S0-BTB-770

Psychiatry

SIXTH EDITION

The House Officer Series is based on Weiner and Levitt's *Neurology for the House Officer*, first published in 1973.

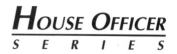

Psychiatry

SIXTH EDITION

David A. Tomb, M.D.

Associate Professor
Department of Psychiatry
University of Utah School of Medicine
Salt Lake City, Utah

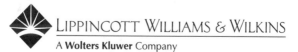

LIPPINCOTT WILLIAMS & WILKINS

A **Wolters Kluwer** Company

Philadelphia · Baltimore · New York · London
Buenos Aires · Hong Kong · Sydney · Tokyo

Acquisitions Editor: Charles W. Mitchell
Developmental Editor: Michael J. D. Standen
Production Editor: Thomas Boyce
Manufacturing Manager: Kevin Watt
Cover Designer: Diana Andrews
Compositor: Circle Graphics
Printer: R R Donnelley

RC
456
T64
1999

© 1999 by LIPPINCOTT WILLIAMS & WILKINS
227 East Washington Square
Philadelphia, PA 19106-3780 USA
LWW.com

All rights reserved. This book is protected by copyright. No part of this book may be reproduced in any form or by any means, including photocopying, or utilized by any information storage and retrieval system without written permission from the copyright owner, except for brief quotations embodied in critical articles and reviews. Materials appearing in this book prepared by individuals as part of their official duties as U.S. government employees are not covered by the above-mentioned copyright.

Printed in the USA

Library of Congress Cataloging-in-Publication Data

Tomb, David A.
    Psychiatry / David A. Tomb. — 6th ed.
        p.   cm. — (House officer series)
    Includes bibliographical references and index.
    ISBN 0-683-30634-0
    1. Psychiatry Handbooks, manuals, etc.   2. Mental illness
Handbooks, manuals, etc.   3. Psychological manifestations of general
diseases Handbooks, manuals, etc.   I. Title.   II. Series.
    [DNLM: 1. Mental Disorders Handbooks.   WM 34 T656pa 1999]
RC456.T64   1999
616.89—dc21
DNLM/DLC
for Library of Congress   99-40550
                                                                            CIP

Care has been taken to confirm the accuracy of the information presented and to describe generally accepted practices. However, the author and publisher are not responsible for errors or omissions or for any consequences from application of the information in this book and make no warranty, expressed or implied, with respect to the currency, completeness, or accuracy of the contents of the publication. Application of this information in a particular situation remains the professional responsibility of the practitioner.

The author and publisher have exerted every effort to ensure that drug selection and dosage set forth in this text are in accordance with current recommendations and practice at the time of publication. However, in view of ongoing research, changes in government regulations, and the constant flow of information relating to drug therapy and drug reactions, the reader is urged to check the package insert for each drug for any change in indications and dosage and for added warnings and precautions. This is particularly important when the recommended agent is a new or infrequently employed drug.

Some drugs and medical devices presented in this publication have Food and Drug Administration (FDA) clearance for limited use in restricted research settings. It is the responsibility of the health care provider to ascertain the FDA status of each drug or device planned for use in their clinical practice.

10 9 8 7 6 5 4 3 2 1

3 3001 00835 3574

Preface

Another four years have passed and it is time for another edition. This time, the driving force is not profound changes in our understanding of the mental illnesses, although there have been a few, but rather an unexpected increase in the number of important new medications available to the practitioner. Over the past half decade, the way we approach both psychotic and mood disorders psychopharmacologically has changed fundamentally and forever. I hope that this new edition adequately reflects those changes. These have not been minor modifications with limited effects but major revisions that provide ways to help a greater number of patients and at less cost in terms of discomfort and side effects.

One additional note: after 20 years and six editions, I would like to (finally) formally thank Bernard I. Grosser, M.D., Chairman of the Department of Psychiatry at the University of Utah School of Medicine for the support and encouragement he has given me over the years to keep this book current and in print. This kind of publishing does not reflect serious research and does not advance one's career or the "glory" of the department. However, he has been unwavering in his support for a succinct and up-to-date volume of this size made available to mental health trainees and young practitioners, and so has given me the freedom to plug away at this book year after year.

David A. Tomb, M.D.

Contents

Chapter 1

Psychiatric Classification

DSM-IV

Psychiatric diagnosis has long been criticized as ambiguous and unreliable. Some diagnoses have been based on subjective, unverifiable, intrapsychic phenomena, whereas others have been heterogeneously broad.

Modern diagnosis attempts to avoid these pitfalls through the use of the 4th edition of the *Diagnostic and Statistical Manual of Mental Disorders* (DSM-IV) (1), which identifies each disorder by a unique specific collection of symptoms. It defines a limited number of identifiable (though possibly overlapping) psychiatric disorders and contains specific diagnostic criteria for each diagnosis. One matches facts from a particular patient's history and clinical presentation with criteria from a likely diagnosis and, if an adequate number are met (a **polythetic** diagnosis; not all the criteria are needed to make the diagnosis), that diagnosis should be made. Each disorder has a unique set of these "operationally defined" diagnostic criteria. Multiple diagnoses are permitted, and each general group of disorders has one disorder "Not Otherwise Specified" (NOS) that allows placement of the (often many) patients who have unusual presentations. In addition, some disorders have **subtypes,** which are mutually exclusive (e.g., *paranoid* schizophrenia) and/or **specifiers** that are not (may change with time, e.g., mild, moderate, and severe, or in full remission). Finally, it is okay to make a **provisional** (you are not sure) or a **deferred** (not enough information) diagnosis.

For example, a patient who (A) has been having delusions and auditory hallucinations that (B) have impaired social relations and functioning at work (C) for at least 6 months and who is without evidence of (D) a general medical condition or (E) prominent symptoms of a major mood disorder must be given the diagnosis of schizophrenia. If the patient also has (F) a flat, inappropriate, or silly affect and (G) disorganized speech and behavior, an additional diagnosis of disorganized subtype should be made.

DSM-IV has improved diagnostic **reliability** (the likelihood that different professionals would make the same diagnosis on the same patient) but has had only a modest impact on **validity** (the certainty that the diagnoses identify unique meaningful conditions). It may well be that DSM-IV has broken psychiatric conditions into too many pieces and that each piece does not represent a "valid" condition (2,3). Note also that DSM-IV makes no assumptions about what causes these disorders (it just describes and categorizes them), and in most cases the etiology is unknown. Although DSM-IV holds up well across cultures, its use in those settings requires special care in the interpretation of symptoms. DSM-IV is far from perfect (4) and thus allows the use of "clinical judgment" as well as strict application of the criteria in making a final diagnosis. And remember, ultimately it is the patient and the patient's narrative/life story we are treating, not the diagnosis.

MULTIAXIAL CLASSIFICATION

In addition to operationally defined criteria, DSM-IV also uses a multiaxial system of classification to capture other important information. A patient is not fully classified until coded on each of five axes (although only the first three axes are needed for an official diagnosis):

- **Axis I:** The clinical disorder(s) described above.
- **Axis II:** Personality disorders and/or mental retardation (none may be present).
- **Axis III:** Physical disorders relevant to the mental disorder.
- **Axis IV:** A listing of psychosocial and environmental *problems,* usually but not always during the preceding year, such as unemployment, divorce, financial problems, victim of child neglect, and so on.
- **Axis V:** The Global Assessment of Functioning Scale (GAF) (DSM-IV p. 32), which is a measure, typically, of *current* gen-

eral functioning but at times of the highest functioning over the preceding year (scale range is 1 to 100) and which is used in treatment planning and predicting outcome.

REFERENCES

1. American Psychiatric Association Task Force on Nomenclature and Statistics. *Diagnostic and statistical manual of mental disorders,* 4th ed. Washington, DC: American Psychiatric Association, 1994.
2. Clark LA, Watson D, Reynolds S. Diagnosis and classification of psychopathology: challenges to the current system and future directions. *Annu Rev Psychol* 1995;46:121–153.
3. Sullivan PF, Kendler KS. Typology of common psychiatric syndromes. *Br J Psychiatry* 1998;173:312–319.
4. Tucker GJ. Putting DSM-IV in perspective. *Am J Psychiatry* 1998; 155: 159–161.

Chapter 2

Assessment

A psychiatric evaluation helps (a) to make a diagnosis, (b) to estimate the severity of the patient's condition, (c) to decide on an initial course of action, (d) to develop a relationship with the patient (therapeutic alliance), (e) to assemble a dynamic understanding of the patient, and (f) to engage the patient in psychotherapy. Some (primarily analytically oriented) psychiatrists argue that the most reliable understanding of a patient results from an open-ended interview in which the course of the interview is directed by the patient's conscious and unconscious concerns. An alternate form of interview, and one encouraged by the requirements of DSM-IV, uses a structured format that demands precise historical and descriptive information and the answers to specific questions (1–4). Which technique produces a more accurate and useful understanding of the patient remains unresolved, yet modern diagnosis requires the structured form described below.

A thorough evaluation of a psychiatric patient consists of a psychiatric history, mental status examination, complete physical examination, laboratory screening evaluation, and, when indicated, specific psychological and biologic tests. The history and mental status are usually obtained during the initial interview.

More is required than merely collecting facts. The interviewer seeks useful information not only from the history and mental status examination but also from the patient's interpersonal style and nonverbal communications and from the sequence and choice of issues raised by the patient. Because there is so much information available from the patient outside the formal part of the interview, it is essential to avoid structuring the interview too early. Initially, allow the patient to express concerns and find out the reason for coming for help (*Why now?*). Be supportive, attentive, nonjudgmental, and encouraging—develop a rapport with the patient and try to get an empathic understanding of his or her distress. Develop a qualitative sense for the patient's impairment. Help allay anxiety, if present. Be patient, friendly, and receptive if the patient is quiet. If the patient rambles, you may have to impose a structure early. If paranoid, progress slowly. Decide early if he or she is likely to be aggressive, suicidal, or in need of hospitalization.

If skillfully conducted, much of the information required by the history and mental status examination may be obtained unobtrusively. As the interview proceeds, you usually can identify and narrow missing data so that more formal questions are minimal. However, certain information is almost always required (e.g., data to satisfy DSM-IV diagnostic criteria, family psychiatric history, or mental status responses to rule out organicity or loss of abstracting ability). At times during the interview, mentally review what is missing and save time toward the end to pursue it by direct questioning. The transition to a more formal style of interviewing can be smooth if rapport has been developed beforehand ("Now I need to ask you some very specific questions").

PSYCHIATRIC HISTORY

Identification of the Patient

1. Name, age, birth date, marital status and children, ethnic status, religion, occupation, education, social class, handicaps, and so on;
2. Identification of informants (if not the patient). Mood and apparent biases of informants;
3. Estimate of the reliability of the information.

Chief Complaint

Usually a verbatim statement of "the problem." Does it differ significantly from the reports of those who accompany the patient?

Present Illness

Usually the focus of the interview. Get the patient's description of and feelings about the illness (problem). Establish the chronologic order of symptoms and treatments. Has the patient noticed any other changes in him or herself? Have there been major life changes during this time or particular stresses and conflicts? Is any secondary gain identifiable? Any *past psychiatric history,* particularly diagnoses and severity of illnesses, types of treatment, or drug use?

Personal History

- **Birth and early development:** Mother's pregnancy and delivery: Prematurity? Planned pregnancy? Get estimate of temperament and behavior problems. Any psychophysiologic problems? (Relatives may be a source of information.)
- **Childhood:** Personality traits, behavior problems, social relationships, school adjustment, family relationships, and family stability. Any abuse or family violence?
- **Social history:** What kind of interpersonal relationships can the patient make? Has he or she been a loner? follower? leader? What kind of group activities has he or she had in the past and in the present? Who are the people important to the patient now? in the past? What was the patient's *premorbid personality?* Military history?
- **Marriage:** At what age? How many times? Relationship patterns within the marriage? Number of children and attitude toward them?
- **Education:** Highest grade attained? Specific academic difficulties? Behavior problems? Social problems?
- **Occupational history:** Concentrate on job changes, length of time jobs have been held, best job obtained and when— get details. Social relations on job; with boss? with workers? How does job compare with ambition? with family expectations?
- **Sexual history:** Sexual orientation? Psychosexual problems or deviant behavior? Feelings about sex?
- **Current social situation:** Personal living situation, income? Social environment? Estimated current marital and family stability and happiness?

Family History

Who lives in the home? The patient should describe them and the relationship with them. Get description of patient's family of origin and his or her role in it. Upwardly mobile family? Get detailed description of psychiatric (and medical) illnesses in family members (*family psychiatric history*).

Medical History

Obtain current and past medical problems and treatments.

MENTAL STATUS EXAMINATION

A mental status examination (5) is a systematic documentation of the quality of mental functioning *at the time of interview.* It helps both with current diagnosis and treatment planning, and it serves as a baseline for future reference. Although much of the information sought in a mental status examination is obtained informally during other parts of the interview, it is usually necessary for the patient to answer a few formal questions if the interviewer is to learn the patient's abilities in each category of mental functioning listed below. Upon concluding the mental status examination, estimate its reliability.

General Presentation

- **Appearance:** Overall impression of the patient: attractive, unattractive, posture, clothes, grooming, healthy versus sickly, old looking versus young looking, angry, puzzled, frightened, ill at ease, apathetic, contemptuous, effeminate, masculine, and so on.
- **General behavior:** Mannerisms, gestures, combative, psychomotor retardation, rigid, twitches, picking, clumsy, hand wringing, and so forth.
- **Attitude toward the examiner:** Cooperative, hostile, defensive, seductive, evasive, ingratiating, and so on.

The psychotic patient may appear disheveled and bizarre with odd posturing (particularly catatonics) and grimacing. Some schizophrenics may stare and others look "blank." Paranoid patients may be hostile and suspicious, borderline patients hostile and angry, whereas histrionic patients often are seductive in manner and dress. Depressed patients may be nearly mute and display psychomotor retardation. Restlessness may suggest anxiety, withdrawal, mania, etc.

State of Consciousness

Is the patient *alert* (e.g., normally aware of both internal and external stimuli) or *hyperalert?* Is the patient *lethargic,* e.g., does he "drift off" or do his thoughts wander? The patient needs to be reasonably alert for the remainder of the examination to be reliable. The causes for decreased alertness are usually organic.

Attention

Can the patient pay attention for short periods of time (*attend*) without being distracted by minor stimuli? Can the patient attend for lengths of time (*concentrate*)? This ability is necessary if you are to assess higher level functions (i.e., they may be intact, but the patient cannot demonstrate them due to lack of attention). Test attention by digit recall (digit span)—e.g., speak a series of numbers in a monotone and ask the patient to repeat them; begin with three numbers and increase by one with each successful trial; a normal maximum is seven numbers repeated. Have them repeat numbers backward; the norm is five. Test concentration by the Random Letter Test—e.g., tell the patient to note (by raising a finger) each time a certain letter is mentioned and then read a long string of letters; most people make very few errors. Defects in attention usually are due to organic causes but may be caused by marked anxiety or psychotic interruption of thoughts.

Speech

Listen to the patient's speech. Is it loud, soft, fast, slow, pressured, mute, etc? Does the patient speak spontaneously? With good vocabulary? Does the patient articulate with difficulty (dysarthria)?

Is there a deficiency in *language* (e.g., aphasia)? This speech is usually identifiable by the experienced listener (e.g., patient tries to communicate but incorrect words are chosen and grammatical errors made) but may be confused with rambling psychotic speech. Manic patients often speak loudly and rapidly; depressed patients are soft and slow. Bizarre speech usually suggests a psychotic and/or organic state.

Orientation

Check for *person* (name? age? when born?), *place* (what place is this? what is your home address?), *time* (today's date? day of the week? time? season?), and *situation* (why are you here?). Time sense is usually the first lost. Major disorientation suggests organicity. Minor loss may reflect temporary stress. If without problems, they are "oriented × 4."

Mood and Affect

Mood is a sustained emotional state (e.g., depressed, euphoric, elevated, anxious, angry, irritable). *Affect* is the patient's current emotional state—it is the state the interviewer can *observe*. Common abnormal affects include flat, blunted, restricted, and inappropriate.

Note whether the affect you observe is consistent with the patient's expressed mood and congruent with thought content. Distinguish a depressed mood from an organically caused apathy. The affective disorders most commonly display alterations in mood but so do psychotic, anxiety (e.g., panic), and organic (e.g., drug use) disorders.

Form of Thought

Does the patient's thinking make sense? Does one thought follow another logically, or does the patient display *circumstantiality* (take forever to make a point; many irrelevant details—overinclusiveness), *flight of ideas* (rapidly jumping from idea to idea; usually stimulated by a previous word or thought but with understandable associations), *evasiveness, loosening of associations* (tangentiality or derailment—thoughts are unrelated, but the patient seems unaware of this), *perseveration* (needless repetition of the same thought or phrase), or *blocking* (speech and train of thought is interrupted and picked up again a few moments or minutes later). Are answers to questions relevant? Ask the patient for impressions of his or her own thoughts. Record quotes of abnormal speech—it adds clarity.

These abnormalities in thought process are most commonly associated with schizophrenic or affective disorders. None are pathognomonic, but any major abnormality suggests a psychotic process.

Thought Content

Check for abnormal preoccupations and obsessions, excessive suspiciousness, phobias, rituals, hypochondriacal symptoms, *déjà vu* experiences, depersonalization, *delusions* (fixed false beliefs—

characterize them as persecutory, of grandeur, of reference, of influence, unsystematized, etc.). *Always* check for preoccupations about suicide or homicide.

Get at the presence of delusions with questions like "Do you have any strong ideas other people don't share?" or "Are there things you think about a lot?"

Delusions usually suggest a functional psychotic disorder (most commonly schizophrenia), but other conditions may display them (e.g., poorly systematized delusions in delirium). Obsessions may occur with psychosis but also are typical of obsessive compulsive disorder. Phobias characterize phobic disorders.

Is the patient unaware that he or she is ill or has abnormal thinking (lacks *insight*)? Does the patient have a generalized loss of ability for *abstractive* thinking (i.e., concreteness)? Test for abstractive ability by

1. **Similarities:** "What do these things have in common?"
   baseball—orange
   car—train
   desk—bookcase
   happy—sad
   horse—apple
2. **Proverbs:** "What do people mean when they say . . . ?"
   When the cat's away, the mice will play.
   The proof of the pudding is in the eating.
   A golden hammer breaks an iron door.
   The tongue is the enemy of the neck.
   The hot coal burns, the cold one blackens.

Always correlate abstractive thinking with intelligence. Concreteness in the face of normal intelligence "suggests" a psychotic thought disorder. Note any bizarre responses to similarities or proverbs—are the answers personalized? Are the answers vague because the patient is aware of failing (e.g., delirium, early dementia) and is obfuscating?

Perceptions

Does the patient display *misperceptions* (draw wrong conclusions from self-evident information)? Are there *illusions* (misinterpretations of sensory stimuli, e.g., a shadow becomes a person) or *hallucinations* (totally imagined sensory perceptions: note whether auditory, visual, tactile, olfactory, etc.)? *Always* determine if hallucinations are accusatory, threatening, or commanding. If not volunteered, detect the presence of hallucinations by questions like "Have you had the experience of walking down the street, hearing your name called, and finding no one there?" or "Have you had any mystical or psychic experiences?"

Illusions are most common in delirium but may also occur in other psychoses. Hallucinations occur in a variety of conditions but most commonly in psychotic disorders. Schizophrenia usually has auditory hallucinations, whereas visual hallucinations are more common in organic conditions. Tactile hallucinations are frequent in sedative-hypnotic and alcohol-withdrawal states.

Judgment

An estimate of the patient's real life problem-solving skills is often difficult to make. Judgment is a complex mental function that depends on maturation of the nervous system (poor in children). The best indicator is usually the patient's behavior, so history is very important. Some sense of the patient's judgment can be obtained through hypothetical examples: "What should you do if you find a stamped, addressed letter?" "What should you do if you lose a book belonging to a library?"

Judgment is regularly impaired in delirium, dementia, psychosis, and some retardation. Its assessment helps determine the patient's capacity for independent functioning.

Memory

Test all three types of memory: immediate (retention and recall), recent, and remote.

Immediate:

1. Digit repetition.
2. Ask the patient to remember three objects and three words—ask for them after 5 minutes (they should be recalled).
3. Ask the patient to count—stop him at 27—(wait 1 minute)—tell him to continue counting—stop at 42—(wait 3 minutes)—then continue counting.

Recent:

1. Ask questions about the past 24 hours (e.g., "How did you travel here?" "What was on the TV news last night?").

Remote:

1. Get personal information such as when were you born? school? work?
2. Ask historical information, for example, name four presidents in this century, the dates of World War II, and so on.

Recent and remote memory usually can be tested inconspicuously during the interview. Is the patient aware of her deficit? What is her attitude toward it? Loss of memory usually indicates an organic process unless it has some of the characteristics of the dissociative disorders (see Chapter 9).

Constructional ability is a sensitive test for early diffuse cortical damage. Draw a diamond and a three-dimensional cube and have the patient copy them. Ask the patient to draw a flowerpot with a flower or the face of a clock set at 2:45. Incomplete or very poorly done responses are suggestive of early organicity.

Intellectual Functioning

Intelligence is a global function that can be estimated from the general tone and content of the interview and by the patient's fund of information and ability to perform calculations.

Fund of knowledge:

How many weeks in a year?
Name the last 6 presidents.
What does the liver do?
How far is it from Chicago to Los Angeles?
Why are light-colored clothes cool?
Who wrote *Remembrances of Things Past?*
What causes rust?
How many nickels in $1.15?

Calculations:

Serial 7's—"take 100 and subtract 7 from it, then take 7 from that answer, etc.";
Serial 3's—"take 3 from 20, etc.";
Simple calculations—$2 \times 3, 5 \times 3, 4 \times 9$.

Calculation relies on functions other than intelligence, including concentration and memory. If in doubt, ask for formal IQ testing. Organic conditions may produce a loss of intellectual functioning, but psychoses seldom do (as long as the patient can concentrate on the tests).

PSYCHOLOGICAL TESTS

Psychological testing is requested for occasional psychiatric patients and may provide a useful enlargement of the understanding of those patients. Although not essential for most patients, testing may

1. Help identify organic syndromes;
2. Help localize organic pathology;
3. Contribute to the identification of borderline psychotic states;
4. Provide a baseline of general and specific functioning;
5. Generally help with differential diagnosis among psychiatric conditions.

Talk to the psychologist. Describe what you are looking for. Ask for recommendations. Although most patients receive a battery of tests, very specific questions may be answered by only one test. Carefully integrate the psychologist's report with your own evaluation but do not allow test results to supersede clinical judgment. Commonly used tests for adults include the following.

Wechsler Adult Intelligence Scale (WAIS): A very useful test. Although it does yield three separate IQ scores (full-scale, verbal, and performance), a careful evaluation of how the patient answered the 11 different subtests within the WAIS provides clues to the presence of a thought disorder, an attention or memory deficit, visual–motor impairment, and so forth.

Minnesota Multiphasic Personality Inventory (MMPI): This is a true–false self-administered personality test of 567 items that takes little of the therapist's time, produces a general description of the patient's personality characteristics, and can even be computer scored. Although a useful global description of the patient, do not stretch it too far diagnostically.

Bender-Gestalt Test: This test is easily administered—the patient draws nine specific geometric figures on a blank sheet of paper. Its greatest application is in detecting visual–motor impairment and organic deficits.

Rorschach Test: This is an unstructured *projective* test that asks the patient to "describe what he sees" in a series of ten standardized ink blots. Elaborate scoring systems exist that allow a skilled examiner to infer elements of the patient's personality functioning. It is used diagnostically to help identify psychoses and personality disorders. Its diagnostic validity, although not ensured, is reasonably high using the standardized rating system devised by Exner.

Thematic Apperception Test (TAT): This is a projective test similar to the Rorschach that draws conclusions from stories a patient generates in response to a series of suggestive but ambiguous human figure drawings.

Draw-a-Person Test: The patient is asked to draw a picture of a "person" and then a picture of a person of the opposite sex. The results are then interpreted by the examiner, usually as a screen for brain damage.

Mini-Mental State Examination (MMSE): A brief, formal, mental status screening examination devised by Folstein (6) for "bedside" use that tests orientation to time and place, immediate and short-term memory, calculation, language, and constructive ability. Although widely used because of its simplicity, it is flawed (7) and improved versions exist.

Psychiatric rating scales are a class of measures that rate emotional symptoms or disorders. They usually consist of lists of short questions that require brief numerical answers and typically are filled out by the patient or the therapist. They serve several purposes: provide a baseline measure of a set of symptoms or diagnoses, allow the severity of psychopathology to be followed longitudinally, complement clinical judgment with an objective measure, evaluate the effectiveness of treatment, provide a uniform standard across evaluators, help determine disposition, and function as a standard measure of patients' symptoms in research trials. They assess differing psychopathology, including general emotional problems [Global Assessment Scale (GAS); Brief Psychiatric Rating Scale (BPRS)], organicity (such as the Folstein MMSE, mentioned above), the diagnosis of mood and psychotic disorders (Schedule for Affective Disorders and Schizophrenia; SADS), depression (Beck Depression Inventory; Hamilton Depression Rating Scale), and anxiety (Hamilton Anxiety Rating Scale; State-Trait Anxiety Scale). There are dozens of rating scales available, and their use is growing rapidly both for their own sake and because managed care agencies increasingly demand objective measures of the severity and course of a patient's illness. Moreover, they are philosophically consistent with the concepts of psychiatric disorder underlying DSM-IV.

ELECTROENCEPHALOGRAM (EEG)

The EEG plays a useful, but only supportive, role in psychiatry. It is suggestive but not definitive in any psychiatric condition, but it does help rule in or out a diversity of conditions. Its primary use is in the differentiation between organic and functional conditions.

1. Epileptics (particularly temporal lobe epilepsy) often mimic "pseudoseizure" psychiatric patients—the EEG helps differentiate (although 30% of epileptics have a normal tracing between attacks).

2. The patient who is confused and disoriented (delirium) due to organic factors usually has diffuse EEG slowing. A major exception is alcohol-withdrawal delirium (delirium tremens), which shows increased fast activity as does confusion due to sedative-hypnotics. Major tranquilizers increase slow wave activity.

3. The patient who has dementia of the Alzheimer type (50% of demented patients) usually has a normal EEG early on, with abnormalities later (a help in staging). Most reversible forms of dementia produce abnormal tracings. The EEG of a person with pseudodementia (e.g., depression that mimics dementia) is usually normal.

4. A variety of organic causes can produce bizarre behavior (e.g., brain tumor, cerebral infarcts, cerebral trauma). A normal EEG does not rule out organic pathology, but an abnormal tracing is suspicious.

Several populations of psychiatric patients have a slightly increased frequency of nonspecific abnormalities on the EEG (e.g., schizophrenics, particularly catatonics, and manic-depressives). Patients with antisocial personality disorder have perhaps the highest frequency of abnormal tracings; look for but do not over-read organic pathology in these patients.

Brain electrical activity topographic mapping (quantitative EEG or QEEG) groups each wavelength type and plots their positions over a map of the head. This new technology may extract more information from EEG data and increase its usefulness. Although still a research tool, it may help diagnose delirium, dementia, and intoxication, as well as stroke, schizophrenia, depression, and obsessive-compulsive disorder (OCD). A related EEG technique, visual and/or auditory evoked potentials (EP), remains a (actively investigated) research tool in psychiatry.

BRAIN IMAGING

Structural Techniques

Both the CT scan and the MRI supply brain structure information useful in psychiatric diagnosis (8). Because it is relatively inexpensive, the CT is used to screen for organic brain disease, particularly in older patients with sudden psychiatric symptoms and in patients with a history of head trauma. The more expensive MRI gives a better image and is much better able to differentiate between gray and white matter and so is used to look for subtle changes in CNS structures and to identify demyelinating disorders, dementia, infarctions, and neoplasms. CT or MRI may be combined with neuropsychological testing or functional imaging like positron emission tomography (PET) or single-photon emission CT (SPECT) for more information.

Functional Techniques

PET and SPECT, both using IV or inhaled radiopharmaceuticals, measure brain metabolic activity (9,10). PET provides better resolution and can provide a direct measure of brain glucose metabolism but is very expensive and available in only a few centers. SPECT is now available in most major medical centers and at a "reasonable" cost but currently reflects brain blood flow and thus is a more indirect measure of metabolism (11). Both remain research techniques, even though they have provided many fascinating, but unproven, insights into psychiatric disorders (e.g., parietal lobe hypofunction may occur in catatonic schizophrenia but not in other types of schizophrenia; inferior right frontal and temporal hypoperfusion is seen in some major depression; orbitofrontal and globus pallidus hyperactivity in OCD). SPECT now has clinical utility in the differential diagnosis of stroke, dementia, and epilepsy and may soon have use in schizo-phrenia, OCD, depression, and brain receptor imaging. In the near future it is likely that PET will teach us much more about the psychobiologic functioning of the brain and SPECT will become a useful diagnostic tool for specific psychiatric conditions.

A noninvasive technique, also available in most major hospitals, is functional MRI (fMRI). It is a sensitive MRI that records local changes in deoxyhemoglobin and presents what is the equivalent of a map of regional blood flow, and thus a map of local neural activity. fMRI is becoming the most readily available and reasonably priced measure of functional brain activity. Other fancy tools, such as magnetoencephalography (MEG), are available in specialized centers.

THE AMYTAL INTERVIEW

The administration of amobarbital (Amytal), thiopental (Pentothal), or pentobarbital (Nembutal) during an interview to produce a sedated state has been used for many years both diagnostically (Amytal interview) and therapeutically (narcoanalysis). Despite a long history of use, the indications for and value of this technique are unclear, and it is currently out of favor.

The technique usually consists of administering 200–500 mg (occasionally more) of sodium amobarbital IV at a rate of 25–50 mg/min. The interviewer talks with the patient throughout administration and halts the drug temporarily when the desired level of sedation is attained (e.g., appearance of lateral nystagmus for light sedation; development of slurred speech for a deeper state). Additional Amytal may be given if the interview is lengthy.

In this sedated state, some patients present a markedly altered clinical picture that may be of diagnostic value. Although opinion varies, diagnostic uses for the Amytal interview may include:

1. Evaluation of mute patients: Patients with *catatonic schizophrenia* often recover dramatically when sedated (although a thought disorder usually remains) but return to the full catatonic state when the Amytal wears off. This helps differentiate catatonia from marked psychomotor retardation in the depressed patient (they show little improvement). Patients mute for other reasons (e.g., hysterical, acute stress) may begin to talk under sedation.
2. *Acute panic states:* Patients immobilized by severe stress may talk about their concerns when sedated and find some relief.
3. *Organic versus functional differentiation:* Patients who are confused, disoriented, or demented due to organic factors usually worsen with Amytal, whereas clinically similar functional patients often clear temporarily.
4. Hysterical phenomena: *Amnesias, fugues,* and *conversion disorders* often are temporarily relieved by Amytal. Useful information may be obtained during this time: e.g., the patient's name and address; the cause of the patient's anger.
5. The interview is less reliably useful with psychotic states (except for catatonic schizophrenia), although some patients may contribute information they wouldn't have otherwise.

Although helpful in confirming some diagnoses, the Amytal interview also may contribute to the treatment of a few patients by allowing them to confront and deal with stressful or troubling experiences which they previously had been reluctant or unable to face. However, the validity of old memories in patients with a presumed past history of child abuse and/or a current dissociative disorder recalled under the Amytal interview is uncertain (the "false memory" versus "repressed memory" controversy).

REFERENCES

1. Carlat DJ. *The psychiatric interview.* Philadelphia: Lippincott Williams & Wilkins, 1999.
2. Morrison J. *The first interview.* New York: Guilford Press, 1993.
3. Othmer E, Othmer SC. *The clinical interview using SDM-IV.* Vol. 1. Washington, DC: American Psychiatric Press, 1994.
4. Shea SC. *Psychiatric interviewing: the art of understanding.* Philadelphia: W.B. Saunders, 1998.
5. Strub RL, Black FW. *The mental status examination in neurology,* 3rd ed. Philadelphia: FA Davis, 1993.
6. Folstein MF, Folstein SE, McHugh PR. "Mini-mental state"—a practical method for grading the mental state of patients for the clinician. *J Am Geriatr Soc* 1975;12:189–198.
7. Wind AW, Schellevis FG, van Staveren G, et al. Limitations of the mini-mental state examination. *Int J Geriatr Psychiatry* 1997;12: 101–108.
8. Soares JC, Mann JJ. The anatomy of mood disorders—review of structural neuroimaging studies. *Biol Psychiatry* 1997;41:86–106.
9. Kennedy SH, Javanmard M, Vaciarino FJ. A review of functional neuroimaging in mood disorders. *Can J Psychiatry* 1997;42:467–475.
10. Orrison WW. 3M Mayneard memorial lecture: functional brain imaging—an overview. *Br J Radiol* 1996;69:493–501.
11. Innis RB. Neuroreceptor imaging with SPECT. *J Clin Psychiatry* 1992;53[Suppl 11]:29–34.

Chapter 3

Psychotic Disorders

Psychosis describes a degree of severity, not a specific disorder. A psychotic patient has a grossly impaired sense of reality, often coupled with emotional and cognitive disabilities, which severely compromises the ability to function. The patient is likely to talk and act in a bizarre fashion, have hallucinations, or strongly hold ideas that are contrary to fact (delusions). He or she may be confused and disoriented and typically is not aware of the impairment (lacks insight).

This chapter covers the major psychotic disorders—i.e., conditions that *must* reach psychotic proportions at some time during their course (although the patients may be nonpsychotic most of the time). Recognize that these are descriptive groupings of clinical syndromes, *not* discrete diseases.

Schizophrenia
  Disorganized type
  Catatonic type
  Paranoid type
  Undifferentiated type
  Residual type
Schizophreniform disorder
Brief psychotic disorder
Schizoaffective disorder
Shared psychotic disorder

Delusional (paranoid) disorder
Psychotic disorder due to a general medical condition
Substance-induced psychotic disorder
Psychotic disorder not otherwise specified (NOS)

Differential Diagnosis

Most psychotic disorders probably have organic bases, although they are unknown. Start by identifying any underlying medical and neurologic causes or psychoses due to substance intoxication or withdrawal. Obtain a complete history and physical on all psychotic patients. Most psychotic disorders present with emotion and thinking disturbances in a patient with a clear sensorium, whereas obviously organic psychoses usually have a degree of delirium (e.g., clouding of consciousness, confusion, disorientation). Unfortunately, exceptions to either pattern are frequent. Possible organic causes of psychosis include almost any type of serious medical illness or drug abuse (see Chapters 5, 6, 14, and 15). Suspect an organic etiology if

- The patient presents with significant memory loss, confusion, disorientation, or clouding of consciousness;
- There is no personal or family history of serious psychiatric illness;
- The patient has a serious medical illness or a chronic medical condition with periodic relapses;
- The psychosis has developed rapidly (e.g., days) in a patient who previously had been functioning well.

Psychiatric conditions that *may* (but don't necessarily) reach psychotic proportions (addressed in other chapters) include:

1. Major depressive disorder or bipolar disorder (see Chapter 4): Look for the psychosis to coexist with and be dominated by an affective component (either manic or depressed) that preceded the development of the psychosis.
2. Brief psychotic disorders may occur with stress in patients with personality disorders of the histrionic, borderline, paranoid, and schizotypal types. Some obsessive-compulsive persons at times may develop a psychosis if they fail to control their environment.
3. Some acute panic or rage attacks may be of psychotic intensity—e.g., rage in the patient with an explosive disorder (see Chapter 7).
4. A few psychotic conditions develop in childhood and continue into the adult years—e.g., **AUTISTIC DISORDER** (DSM-IV p. 66, 299.00) and **PERVASIVE DEVELOPMENTAL DISORDER NOS** (DSM-IV p. 77, 299.80).

5. Psychotic states occasionally may be mimicked unconsciously or even "faked": Factitious Disorder with Predominantly Psychological Signs and Symptoms; Malingering.

SCHIZOPHRENIA

Schizophrenia is the most common psychotic disorder; almost 1% of people worldwide develop it during their lifetime and over 2 million persons are affected in the United States. It occurs more frequently in urban populations and in lower socioeconomic groups, probably due to a "downward drift" (i.e., poorly functional unemployable persons end up in marginal settings). Poor environments do not "cause" the disorder, although they make it more intractable.

The diagnosis of schizophrenia has had a checkered history. There have been many different ways to make the diagnosis, which have thus represented different populations of patients. The current diagnostic scheme (DSM-IV) uses specific objective criteria to define several forms of schizophrenia. Because there are no pathognomonic findings, "schizophrenia" is a *clinical* diagnosis that may represent a nonspecific syndrome of heterogeneous etiologies. However, biologic, genetic, and phenomenologic information suggest that it is a valid disorder(s). The five identified subtypes are also based on clinical variables.

Clinical Presentation

Although the nature of schizophrenia is uncertain, the current clinical description and method of making the diagnosis are more clear (DSM-IV).

Most schizophrenics are psychotic for only a small part of their lives. Typically they spend many years in a **residual phase** during which time they display minor features of their illness. During these residual periods, patients may be withdrawn, isolated, and "peculiar." They usually are noticeable to others and may lose their jobs or friends both because of their own lack of interest and ability to perform and because they behave oddly. Their thinking and speech are vague and are believed by others to be odd and to "not quite make sense." They may be convinced that they are different from others, believe that they have special powers and sensitivities, and have "mystical" or "psychic" experiences. Their personal appearance and manners deteriorate, and they may display affect that is blunted, flat, or inappropriate. Although they maintain close to normal intelligence, performance on most cognitive tests is modest. They are frequently anhedonic (unable to experience pleasure). Often this deterioration merely represents a gradual worsening of a condition the patient has displayed for many years—the first psychotic episode may have been preceded by a similar period of eccentric thinking and behavior (**prodromal phase**).

A **prepsychotic personality** is seen in some chronic schizophrenics and is characterized by social withdrawal, social awkwardness, and marked shyness in a youth who has difficulty in school despite a normal IQ. An equally common pattern is involvement in minor antisocial activities in the year or two before the initial psychotic episode. Many of these patients have previously received the diagnosis of schizoid, borderline, antisocial, or schizotypal personality disorder. It is only when they develop their first psychotic episode [normally in their teens or early 20s (men) or 20s and early 30s (women); a first "breakdown" after age 40 is unusual] that the diagnosis is changed to schizophrenia. Often a presumed precipitating stress can be identified. The typical **acute psychosis** displays a variable mixture of several of the following symptoms.

Disturbance of Thought Form

These patients usually have a **formal thought disorder,** i.e., their thinking is frequently incomprehensible to others and appears illogical. Characteristics include

- **Loosening of associations** (derailment or tangential associations): Patients' ideas are disconnected. They may jump obliviously from topic to unconnected topic, confusing the listener. When this occurs frequently (e.g., in midsentence), the speech is often incoherent.
- **Overinclusiveness:** Patients continually may disrupt the flow of their thoughts by including irrelevant information.
- **Neologisms:** Patients coin new words (which may have a symbolic meaning for them).
- **Blocking:** Speech is halted (often in midsentence) and then picked up a moment (or minutes) later, usually at another place. This may represent the patients' ideas being interrupted

by intrusive thoughts (e.g., hallucinations). These patients are often very distractible and have a short attention span.

- **Clanging:** Patients choose their next words and themes based on the sound of the words they have just used rather than the thought content (e.g., "Yesterday I went to the store." The patient looks around and then says, "I guess I'd better clean the floor.").
- **Echolalia:** Patients repeat words or phrases in a musical or singsong fashion but without an apparent effort to communicate.
- **Concreteness:** Patients of normal or above average IQ think in abstract terms poorly.
- **Alogia:** Patients may speak very little (but without being intentionally resistant; *poverty of speech*) or may speak a normal amount but say very little (*poverty of speech content*).

Disturbance of Thought Content

Delusions are fixed false beliefs far beyond credibility that may be "bizarre" (e.g., "my right eye is a computer that controls the world") or "nonbizarre" (just very unlikely; "the FBI follows me") and remain unmodified despite clear evidence to the contrary. They are common in most serious mental disorders, but some specific forms of delusional thought are particularly frequent in schizophrenia. The more acute the psychosis, the more likely the delusion is to be disorganized and nonsystematized:

- *Bizarre confused delusions;*
- *Persecutory delusions,* particularly nonsystematic types;
- *Grandiose delusions;*
- *Delusions of influence*—patients believes they can control events through telepathy;
- *Delusions of reference*—patients are convinced of "meanings" behind events and people's actions that are directed specifically toward themselves;
- *Delusions of thought broadcasting*—the belief that others can hear the patients' thoughts;
- *Delusions of thought insertion*—the belief that someone else's thoughts have been inserted into the patients' minds.

Many schizophrenic patients display *lack of insight* (1), that is, the patient is unaware of his or her own illness or of his or her need for treatment, even though the disorder is evident to others.

Disturbance of Perception

Most common are **hallucinations,** usually auditory but also visual, olfactory, and tactile. Auditory hallucinations (most often voices—one or several) may include a running commentary about the patient and events, derogatory or threatening comments made to the patient, or direct orders to the patient (command hallucinations). The voices often (but not necessarily) are perceived as coming from outside the patient's head, and occasionally the patient may hear his or her own thoughts spoken aloud (often to his or her shame or embarrassment). The voices are quite real to the patient, except in the early phases of the psychosis.

These patients may also have illusions, depersonalizations (feels like they are observing themselves from the outside), derealizations (the world seems unreal), and a hallucinatory sense of bodily change.

Disturbance of Emotions

Acutely psychotic patients may display various emotions and may switch from one to another in a surprisingly short span of time. Three frequent (but not pathognomonic) underlying affects are

- **Blunted or flat affect:** The patient expresses very little emotion, even when it is appropriate to do so. He may appear to be without warmth.
- **Inappropriate affect:** The affect may be intense, but it is inconsistent with the patient's thoughts or speech.
- **Labile affect:** Marked changes in affect over a short period of time.

Disturbance of Behavior

Many different bizarre and inappropriate behaviors may be seen, including strange grimacing and posturing, ritual behavior, excessive silliness, aggressiveness, and some sexual inappropriateness.

An acute psychotic attack can last weeks or months (occasionally years). Many patients have recurrences of the active phase periodically throughout their lives, typically separated by months or years. During the intervening periods, patients usually present residual symptoms (often with the degree of impairment gradually increasing over the years); however, a few patients are symptom free between acute episodes. Many schizophrenic patients in remission display early signs of a developing relapse—always look for them. These early signs include increasing restlessness and nervousness, loss of appetite, mild depression and anhedonia, insomnia, and trouble concentrating.

Classification

To be considered schizophrenic, a patient must (DSM-IV p. 285)

1. have had at least *6 months* of
2. sufficiently *deteriorated* occupational, interpersonal, and self-supportive functioning;
3. have been *actively psychotic* in a characteristic fashion during at least part of that period; and
4. must not be able to account for the symptoms by the presence of a schizoaffective or major mood disorder, autism, or an organic condition.

The *course* of the illness should be classed as continuous, episodic with or without interepisode residual symptoms, or single episode in partial or full remission. Moreover, all schizophrenic patients should be classed as one of five recognized subtypes that describes the most frequently occurring behavioral manifestations of the illness. There have been numerous subclassifications of schizophrenia in the past, all unsatisfactory, and the current divisions share some of those deficiencies. Although genetic data suggest that schizophrenia is a fairly stable diagnosis (2), there is no comparable information for the subtypes. Symptomatically, they tend to overlap, and the diagnosis can shift from one to another with time (either during one episode or in a subsequent episode). Finally, over the years, the clinical presentations of many patients tend to converge toward a common picture of interpersonal withdrawal, flattened affect, idiosyncratic thinking, and impaired social and personal functioning. (At the same time, the course becomes more stable, with fewer acute symptoms or episodes.)

Disorganized Type (DSM-IV p. 288, 295.10)

The patient has (A) blunted, silly, or inappropriate affect, (B) frequent incoherence, and (C) no systematized delusions. Grimacing and bizarre mannerisms are common.

Catatonic Type (DSM-IV p. 289, 295.20)

The patient may have any one (or a combination) of several forms of catatonia:

1. **Catatonic stupor or mutism:** Patient does not appreciably respond to the environment or to the people in it. Despite appearances, these patients are often thoroughly aware of what is going on around them.
2. **Catatonic negativism:** Patient resists all directions or physical attempts to move him or her.
3. **Catatonic rigidity:** Patient is physically rigid.
4. **Catatonic posturing:** Patient assumes bizarre or unusual postures.
5. **Catatonic excitement:** Patient is extremely (e.g., wildly) active and excited. May be life-threatening (e.g., due to exhaustion).

Paranoid Type (DSM-IV p. 287, 295.30)

This is the most stable, and most common (3), subtype over time and usually develops later than other forms of schizophrenia. The patient must display consistent, often paranoid, delusions that he or she may or may not act on. These patients are often uncooperative and difficult to deal with and may be aggressive, angry, or fearful, but they are less likely to display disorganized incoherent behavior.

Undifferentiated Type (DSM-IV p. 289, 295.90)

The patient has prominent hallucinations, delusions, and other evidence of active psychosis (e.g., confusion, incoherence) but without the more specific features of the preceding three categories.

Residual Type (DSM-IV p. 290, 295.60)

The patient is in remission from active psychosis but displays symptoms of the residual phase (e.g., social withdrawal, flat or inappropriate affect, eccentric behavior, loosening of associations, and illogical thinking).

Prognosis

Schizophrenia is a chronic disorder. A person gradually may become more withdrawn, "eccentric," and nonfunctional over many years. Some patients may experience low-level delusions and hallucinations indefinitely. Many of the more dramatic and acute symptoms disappear with time, but the patient ends up chronically needing sheltered living or spending years in mental hospitals. Involvement with the law for misdemeanors is common (e.g., vagrancy, disturbing the peace) as is associated mixed drug abuse. A few patients become somewhat demented. Overall life expectancy is shortened, primarily due to accidents, suicide, and an inability of the patients to care for themselves.

This pattern has exceptions. Psychiatrists have long distinguished between *process* schizophrenia (slowly developing; chronic deteriorating course) and *reactive* schizophrenia (rapid onset; somewhat better prognosis). Likewise, they have differentiated between **positive symptoms** (hallucinations, delusions, bizarre behavior, etc.), which frequently respond to usual antipsychotic medications, and **negative symptoms** (flattened affect, poverty of speech, anhedonia, social withdrawal, etc.), which don't (although the newer antipsychotics may break this rule). Clinical characteristics associated with an improved prognosis include (4)

1. A rapid onset of the active psychotic symptoms;
2. An onset after age 30, particularly in women;
3. Good premorbid social and occupational functioning. Past performance remains the best predictor of future performance;
4. Marked confusion and emotional features during the acute episode (positive symptoms); some question this;
5. A probable precipitating stress to the acute psychosis and no evidence of CNS abnormalities;
6. No family history of schizophrenia.

Process and reactive forms of schizophrenia may be etiologically (and biologically?) distinct. Although there is great variability, Disorganized type generally has the worst prognosis, whereas Paranoid type (and some catatonics) have the best. The prognosis is worsened if the patient abuses drugs (5) or lives in a dysfunctional family setting.

About 25%–50% of patients recovering from an acute episode develop a major depression during the months after improvement (*postpsychotic depression*). Although treatment resistant, psychotherapy and antidepressant medication may be useful (lithium and/or anticonvulsants may also help). Watch for it—the suicide rate is increased in this population [particularly in patients aware of the seriousness of their illness (6)]—but don't overdiagnose because some of these patients may have a medication-induced akinesia, mimicking depression.

Biology

No pathognomonic structural or functional abnormality has been found in schizophrenics; however, numerous intriguing abnormalities exist (and have been replicated, as well as contested) in subpopulations of patients. The most generally accepted abnormalities include stable *lateral and third ventricular enlargements* (7) that seem to precede the onset of the illness; *bilateral atrophy of the medial temporal lobes* (8) and specifically of the amygdala and the hippocampal and parahippocampal gyri; *spacial disorientation of the hippocampal pyramidal cells* (9); and *decreased volume of the dorsolateral prefrontal cortex*. These changes all appear static and seem to have been present from about the time of birth (no gliosis) in some studies (10) and show progression in others. Their locations are suggestive of the behavioral disturbances found in schizophrenia; e.g., hippocampal abnormalities may be associated with memory impairment and frontal lobe atrophy may account for the negative symptoms of schizophrenia. Other less well-confirmed findings include CSF cytomegalovirus antibodies, P-type (stimulated) atypical lymphocytes, abnormal left hemisphere function, impaired transmission in and reduced size of the corpus callosum, a small cerebellar vermis, decreased frontal lobe blood flow and glucose metabolism (by PET), EEG and auditory P300 EP abnormalities (by QEEM), difficulty focusing attention, and slowed reaction time, to name a few. Also, among individuals who develop schizophrenia, there is an increased incidence of birth complications (10) (prematurity, low birth weight, birth during an influenza epidemic), a greater likelihood to have been born in the late winter and early spring, and minor neurologic abnormalities. The significance of these findings is unknown. However, taken together, they underscore (a) the biologic nature and (b) the heterogeneity of schizophrenia.

Biochemistry

The biochemical etiology of schizophrenia is unknown. Most major hypotheses implicate an abnormality of central neurotransmitters. The best researched theory postulates excessive central dopamine activity (the *dopamine hypothesis*) and is based on three key findings:

1. The antipsychotic activity of neuroleptic medications (e.g., phenothiazines) is derived in major part from their blockade of postsynaptic dopamine receptors (of the D_2 type).
2. Amphetamine psychosis often is clinically indistinguishable from an acute paranoid schizophrenic psychosis. Amphetamines release central dopamine. Also, amphetamines worsen schizophrenia.
3. There is an increased number of D_2 receptors in the caudate nucleus, nucleus accumbens, and putamen in schizophrenics.

Studies of the D_1, D_3, and D_4 receptors have been, as yet, unproductive (11). Other theories include elevated CNS serotonin (and particularly 5-HT_{2A} receptors) and excessive limbic forebrain NE (occurs in some schizophrenics and decreases with medication and improved clinical state).

Genetics

Schizophrenia has a significant inherited component: complex and polygenic (12). According to *consanguinity studies,* schizophrenia is a familial disorder (i.e., "runs in families"). The closer the relative, the greater the risk. In *twin studies* (13), monozygotic twins are 4–6 times more likely to develop illness than dizygotes. In *adoption studies,* children of schizophrenic parents adopted away at birth into normal families have the same increased rate of illness as if they had been raised by their natural parents (Table 3.1).

Several nonpsychotic disorders occur with increased frequency in the families of schizophrenics and may be related

TABLE 3.1   Genetic Counseling—Lifetime Risk of Developing Schizophrenia

General population	1%
Monozygotic twins[a]	40–50%
Dizygotic twins	10%
Sibling of schizophrenic	10%
Parent of schizophrenic	5%
Child of one schizophrenic parent	10–15%
Child of two schizophrenic parents	30–40%

[a] Note that 50% of monozygotic twins *do not* both develop schizophrenia; thus, clearly environment plays a role. Development of illness reflects nature *and* nurture.

genetically: schizotypal and borderline personality disorders (the *schizophrenia spectrum disorders*), obsessive-compulsive disorder, and possibly antisocial and paranoid personality disorders.

Modern molecular genetic research, primarily chromosomal linkage studies, has found nothing definitive. The strongest evidence points to chromosome 6, yet the expert consensus is that schizophrenia is genetically and environmentally multifactorial.

Family Processes

Family dynamics and turbulence play a major role in producing a relapse or maintaining a remission. Patients who are discharged to home are more likely to relapse over the following year than are those who are placed in a residential setting. Most at risk are patients from hostile families or families that display excessive anxiety, overconcern, or overprotectiveness toward the patient (called *expressed emotion*) (14). Schizophrenic patients often do not "emancipate" from their families.

Some researchers have identified peculiar and pathologic styles of communication in these families; typically, communications are vague and subtly illogical. In 1956, Bateson (15) described a characteristic "double bind" in which the patient is frequently required by a key family member to respond to an overt message that contradicts a covert message. However, recent work suggests that these family communication patterns are as likely to be the effect of having a schizophrenic child as the cause of it.

Differential Diagnosis

Schizophrenia must be differentiated from all those conditions that produce active psychoses (see above). Of all the possibilities, be particularly careful to eliminate schizoaffective disorder, the major affective disorders, and several organic conditions that may closely mimic schizophrenia, e.g., early Huntington's chorea, early Wilson's disease, temporal lobe epilepsy, frontal or temporal lobe tumors, early MS, early SLE, porphyria, general paresis, chronic drug use, chronic alcoholic hallucinosis, and the adult form of metachromatic leukodystrophy. Carefully evaluate catatonia for medical/neurologic conditions.

Treatment

Biologic Methods (see Chapter 23)

Treat acute psychoses with antipsychotics, preferably the new "atypical" antipsychotics (equivalent dose range = chlorpromazine 300–600 mg/day; occasionally more). Low-dose antipsychotic drug maintenance is the norm; after the first relapse, maintenance medication usually should be continued for years. Because noncompliance is common (particularly among substance abusers), long-acting depot fluphenazine or haloperidol may be the drug of choice for many patients. Traditional antipsychotics are primarily useful in controlling the positive symptoms, whereas several of the newer atypicals help with negative symptoms as well (16). Be aware that a protracted excessive dose may chronically hinder patient functioning. A subgroup of schizophrenics may benefit from augmentation with either lithium or a benzodiazepine (particularly in agitated or anxious patients, e.g., diazepam 15–30+ mg/day or clonazepam 5–15 mg/day).

The new gold standard is clozapine (Clozaril), an expensive, dangerous (unpredictable, potentially lethal agranulocytosis), effective antipsychotic that clinically improves and is better received (due to fewer side effects) by 1/3 or more of refractory chronic patients. It can be used safely with *uninterrupted* weekly monitoring of WBC counts. Use it after other serious antipsychotic trials have failed (not a "first run" drug), but BE SURE YOU MONITOR CLOSELY.

ECT may be useful for rapid control of a few acute psychotics. Very few chronic schizophrenics who respond poorly to medication may improve with ECT—unpredictable.

Psychosocial Methods

The primary mode of treatment of schizophrenia is pharmacologic. Long-term insight psychotherapy has a limited place. On the other hand, supportive reality-oriented psychosocial methods are particularly useful in the long-term treatment of schizophrenia.

The acutely psychotic patient should be approached cautiously, but *should* be approached. Keep a comfortable distance from the patient if he appears disturbed by your presence. It is essential to establish some communication with these patients.

1. Talk to the patient. Be relaxed, interested, and supportive. Give the impression that you believe the patient can respond appropriately to you.
2. Be specific. Ask pointed factual questions. Try to identify the patient's major current fears and concerns but do not be led into a lengthy discussion of complex delusions and hallucinations.
3. Take your time during the interview. Don't rush the patient to respond to each question but do maintain some control over the direction of the conversation.
4. Make some specific observations of the patient's behavior (e.g., "you look frightened"; "you look angry") but do not become involved in lengthy "interpretations." Don't draw incorrect conclusions about the patient's emotional state from inappropriate affect.
5. Explain to the patient what is being done to him or her, and why.
6. If the conversation is going nowhere (e.g., the patient refuses to talk), break off the interview with a positive expectation (e.g., "I'll be back to see you in a little while when you are feeling better and are able to talk").

If the acutely psychotic patient is delirious, suicidal, homicidal, and/or has no community support, hospitalize. It is usually better to avoid long-term hospitalization if alternate outpatient arrangements are possible: The deleterious effects of chronic hospitalization are real (regression and marked withdrawal, loss of skills, etc.). The recent trend has been toward short hospital stays during acute episodes with maintenance as outpatients in between.

When hospitalized, allow the patient as much independence as his or her behavior permits within the limits of a safe environment. *Therapeutic milieus* (e.g., therapeutic community, token economy, etc.) all depend on community support (staff *and* patients)—be aware of the patient's behavior and provide helpful "corrective feedback." The milieu is a place for the patient to develop skills in maintaining interpersonal relationships and to learn new methods of coping. *Behavior modification* has been found clearly effective at eliminating specific unacceptable behaviors and in teaching low-level personal skills with some regressed, poorly functioning inpatients.

Most schizophrenics can be treated as outpatients. Several principles should be kept in mind.

- See the patient frequently enough to safely monitor medication and detect early deterioration (e.g., weekly, monthly, or even every several months—depending on the patient's course and reliability).
- Communicate with the patient clearly and unambiguously. Be factual and goal oriented. Avoid extensive discussion of hallucinations and delusions (although a recent study suggests that using cognitive therapy to change what the patient thinks of the voices may decrease their frequency). Help the patient with reality issues (e.g., living arrangements, work). Help the patient avoid excessive stress. Recognize that the more productive and skillful the patient, the more likely he or she is to maintain a recovery—encourage the patient to hold an *appropriate* job. Provide *social skills training* (17).
- Talk about medication (e.g., the need for it, the patient's feelings about taking it, etc.).
- Develop a consistent trusting relationship (often difficult). Be empathic over time, even when the patient is being "unreasonable," but also maintain a professional distance. Be a constant presence.
- Learn the patient's strengths and weaknesses. Teach him to identify an impending decompensation. What are the precipitants, if any? If the patient misses appointments, investigate (he may be relapsing). If the patient is decompensating, be ready to insist on hospitalization. Recognize that overstimulation and overindependence can precipitate a decompensation. These patients are at risk for suicide at times during their illnesses (particularly if they have self-destructive command hallucinations).
- Always evaluate the family. Have they contributed to the patient's decompensation? Can the members deal appropriately with the patient's illness? Are they hostile? Suspicious? Overprotective? Consider *family therapy*—reality-based, in-home, family/patient interventions may be particularly useful. Family members often need considerable support and understanding themselves. When worked with well, they can be a (the?) major help to the patient.
- Consider *group therapy*. The usual orientation is toward support and reality testing. It helps with resocialization, forces interpersonal interactions, and provides support. Several studies have shown it to be effective (in combination with medication) in preventing relapse in outpatients.

- Know and use community resources. Be alert to the devastating effect on the patient of a poor quality of life (e.g., does he live in a "psychiatric ghetto" or "on the street?").
- Do not expect too much. Many patients have chronic disability.

SCHIZOPHRENIFORM DISORDER (DSM-IV p. 291, 295.40)

This disorder is clinically indistinguishable from brief psychotic disorder and schizophrenia except that the symptoms last more than 1 month but less than 6 months. This population of patients seems to differ from schizophrenic patients in several important ways:

1. Symptoms begin and end more abruptly;
2. Symptoms are usually more turbulent and "acute";
3. There is good premorbid adjustment and higher functioning after recovery;
4. There is only a slightly increased prevalence of schizophrenia in the family. There may be a higher prevalence of affective disorder.

Thus, schizophreniform disorder appears to be a separate disease from schizophrenia. Recognize, however, that many schizophrenic patients pass through a period (i.e., the first 6 months) when their diagnosis needs to be schizophreniform disorder. Also, don't miss an organic psychosis.

Treatment is similar to that of an acute schizophrenic episode, but the prognosis is better (18).

BRIEF PSYCHOTIC DISORDER (DSM-IV p. 304, 298.8)

This condition describes those patients who experience an acute psychotic episode lasting longer than 1 day but less than 1 month and that may ["with marked stressor(s)"] or may not ["without marked stressor(s)"] immediately follow an important life stress or ("with postpartum onset") a pregnancy. The illness comes as a surprise—there is usually no forewarning that the person is likely to break down, although this disorder is more common in people with a preexisting personality disorder (particularly histrionic and borderline types).

The psychosis is typically very turbulent and dramatic with marked emotional lability, bizarre behavior, confused and incoherent speech, transient disorientation and memory loss, and/or brief but striking hallucinations and delusions. Thus, it mimics the acute psychotic onset of a major affective disorder, schizophreniform disorder, or psychosis with delirium. *Always* carefully rule out medical conditions and particularly substance-induced problems. The validity of this diagnosis as a separate category is debated.

Treat the acutely psychotic patient with understanding, a secure environment, and antipsychotic medication, if needed. The patient usually recovers completely in several days, and the long-term prognosis is good, although the patient may be at risk for future brief episodes when equivalently stressed.

SCHIZOAFFECTIVE DISORDER (DSM-IV p. 295, 295.70)

This is a vague and poorly defined disorder meant for patients who have evidence of *both* schizophrenia and major affective disorder with depressed mood. These patients may present with an affective disturbance that grades into a purely schizophrenic picture or may display symptoms of both conditions simultaneously, although the schizophrenic symptoms dominate. It is a genetically heterogeneous disorder—both schizophrenia and mood disorders occur with increased frequency in family members. Be cautious that you do not mistake it for a substance-induced psychosis [e.g., amphetamines, phencyclidine (PCP), or exogenous steroids]. Much work remains to be done to better define these patients.

Treat as one would the equivalent schizophrenic or affective patient. Antipsychotics are generally most useful, but lithium has benefitted some patients. These patients seem to have a better prognosis than those with schizophrenia but a poorer outcome than those with a mood disorder (19).

DELUSIONAL DISORDER (DSM-IV p. 301, 297.1)

These patients *do not* display the pervasive disturbances of mood and thought found in other psychotic conditions. They do not have flat or inappropriate affect, prominent hallucinations, or markedly bizarre delusions. They *do* have one or more delusions, often of persecution but also of infidelity, grandiosity, somatic change, or erotomania that are

1. Usually specific (e.g., involve a certain person or group, a given place or time, or a particular activity);
2. Usually well organized (e.g., the "culprits" have elaborate reasons for what they are doing, which the patient can detail);
3. Usually grandiose (e.g., a powerful group is interested just in *them*);
4. Not bizarre enough to suggest schizophrenia.

These patients (who tend to be in their 40s) may be unrecognizable until their delusional system is pointed out by family or friends. Even then the diagnosis may be difficult because they may be too mistrustful to confide in the examiner and don't voluntarily seek treatment. They are frequently hypersensitive, argumentative, and litigious and come to attention through ill-founded legal activities. Although they may perform well occupationally and in areas distant from their delusions, they tend to be social isolates either by preference or as a result of their interpersonal inhospitality (e.g., spouses frequently abandon them). Social and occupational dysfunction, when it occurs, usually is in direct response to their delusions.

These conditions appear to form a clinical continuum with conditions like paranoid personality disorder and paranoid schizophrenia; delineation of the limits of each syndrome awaits further research. Rule out an affective disorder—morbid jealousy and paranoid ideas are common in depression. Paranoia is common among the elderly (20) (see Chapter 24) and among stimulant drug abusers. Acute paranoid reactions frequently are seen in patients with mild delirium and in patients who are bedridden (and sensory deprived).

Etiology is unknown. No genetic or biologic factors have been identified. There is a higher incidence among refugee and minority groups and among those with impaired hearing. There is a tendency for their family relationships to be characterized by turbulence, callousness, and coldness, yet the significance of this pattern is unclear. Typical defense mechanisms seen in these patients include denial, projection, and regression.

Treatment

Treatment is notoriously difficult (21). Individual psychotherapy is useful. Emphasis should be on developing a trusting relationship, with the patient seeing the therapist as neutral and accepting. Interfere with the patient's freedom of choice as little as possible. Gradually help the patient see his or her world from your perspective. These patients are *very* sensitive to criticism (overt or implied), so this kind of a relationship is extremely difficult to develop and maintain.

Antipsychotic medication may help a few—it may at least take the energy out of the delusion. Antidepressants appear promising—consider them.

SHARED PSYCHOTIC DISORDER (DSM-IV p. 306, 297.3)

An otherwise normal person may adopt the delusional system of someone else. Most commonly, a dependent isolated wife will accept the delusional ideas of her (dominant) spouse (e.g., both may come to believe that their children are attempting to murder them with poison gas). When *two* people share equally the same delusion, it is *folie à deux*. Separation of the partners with shared delusions often results in disappearance of the delusions in the healthier member.

PSYCHOTIC DISORDER DUE TO A GENERAL MEDICAL CONDITION (DSM-IV p. 309, 293.81 OR 293.82)

These patients have a medical condition that *causes* prominent delusions (293.81) or hallucinations (293.82) about which they have no insight and cannot appreciate the symptom's connection to their medical illness. Of course, a careful medical workup is in order, and even then the relation between the psychosis and the medical condition is often uncertain. Look for medical symptoms that appear just after the onset or worsening of the medical problem, prominent visual or olfactory hallucinations, and/or the "wrong age" of onset for normal psychoses (e.g., often in the elderly). Many conditions can produce an isolated psychosis (see Chapters 14 and 15): Don't use this diagnosis if symptoms occur only in the presence of an illness-related delirium or dementia.

SUBSTANCE-INDUCED PSYCHOTIC DISORDER (DSM-IV p. 314)

Drugs of abuse, certain medications (see Chapter 13), and toxins all can occasionally produce flagrant psychoses, usually with marked organic features such as confusion and prominent visual, olfactory, or tactile hallucinations. Most drugs of abuse can produce temporary psychoses with intoxication, whereas a few (e.g., alcohol and hypnotic-sedatives) produce them upon withdrawal in the dependent patient (see Chapters 16 and 17). Most intoxication psychoses resolve upon discontinuing the drug but occasionally may persist if caused by heavy use of stimulants, PCP, or LSD.

PSYCHOTIC DISORDER NOS (DSM-IV p. 315, 298.9)

If a psychotic patient does not have an affective disorder, an organic condition, or one of the disorders in this chapter and is not malingering, he or she has psychotic disorder NOS. The most common use of this classification is for patients for whom there is insufficient information to make a more specific diagnosis.

REFERENCES

1. Young DA, Zakzanis KK, Bailey C, et al. Further parameters of insight and neuropsychological deficit in schizophrenia and other chronic mental disease. *J Nerv Ment Dis* 1998;186:44–50.
2. Chen YR, Swann AC, Burt DB. Stability of diagnosis in schizophrenia. *Am J Psychiatry* 1996;153:682–686.
3. Tateyama M, Kudo I, Hashimoto M, et al. Is paranoid schizophrenia the most common subtype? *Psychopathology* 1999;32:98–106.
4. Wieselgren IM, Lindstrom LH. A prospective 1–5 year outcome study in first-admitted and readmitted schizophrenic patients. *Acta Psychiatr Scand* 1996;93:9–19.
5. Gupta S, Hendricks S, Kenkel AM, et al. Relapse in schizophrenia: is there a relationship to substance abuse? *Schizophr Res* 1996;20:153–156.
6. Amador XF, Friedman JH, Kasapis C, et al. Suicidal behavior in schizophrenia and its relationship to awareness of illness. *Am J Psychiatry* 1996;153:1185–1188.
7. Gur RE, Cowell P, Turetsky BI, et al. A follow-up magnetic resonance imaging study of schizophrenia. *Arch Gen Psychiatry* 1998;55:145–152.
8. Nelson MD, Saykin AJ, Flashman LA, et al. Hippocampal volume reduction in schizophrenia as assessed by magnetic resonance imaging. *Arch Gen Psychiatry* 1998;55:433–440.
9. Conrad AJ, Abebe T, Austin R, et al. Hippocampal pyramidal cell disarray in schizophrenia as a bilateral phenomenon. *Arch Gen Psychiatry* 1991;48:413–417.
10. Buka SL, Goldstein JM, Seidman LJ, et al. Prenatal complications, genetic vulnerability, and schizophrenia. *Psychiatric Ann* 1999;29:151–156.

11. Kerwin RW, Collier D. The dopamine D4 receptor in schizophrenia: an update. *Psychol Med* 1996;26:221–227.

12. Tsuang MT, Gilbertson MW, Faraone SV. The genetics of schizophrenia: current knowledge and future research. *Schizophr Res* 1991;4: 157–171.

13. Cannon TD, Kaprio J, Lönnqvist J, et al. The genetic epidemiology of schizophrenia in a Finnish twin cohort. *Arch Gen Psychiatry* 1998;55: 67–74.

14. Butzlaff RL, Hooley JM. Expressed emotion and psychiatric relapse. *Arch Gen Psychiatry* 1998;55:547–552.

15. Bateson G, Jackson DD, Haley J, Weakland JH. Towards a theory of schizophrenia. *Behav Sci* 1956;1:251–256.

16. Schooler NR. Negative symptoms in schizophrenia: assessment of the effect of risperidone. *J Clin Psychiatry* 1994;55[Suppl 5]:22–28.

17. Penn DL, Mueser KT. Research update on the psychosocial treatment of schizophrenia. *Am J Psychiatry* 1996;153:607–617.

18. Benazzi F. DSM-III-R schizophreniform disorder with good prognostic features: a six-year follow-up. *Can J Psychiatry* 1998;43:180–182.

19. Strakowski SM, Keck PE, Sax KW, et al. Twelve-month outcome of patients with DSM-III-R schizoaffective disorder. *Schizophr Res* 1999; 35:167–174.

20. Yassa R, Suranyi-Cadotte B. Clinical characteristics of late-onset schizophrenia and delusional disorder. *Schizophr Bull* 1993;19:701–707.

21. Lane RD. Successful fluoxetine treatment of pathological jealousy. *J Clin Psychiatry* 1990;51:345–346.

Chapter 4

Mood Disorders

Patients with disorders of mood are common (3%—5% of the population at any one time) and are seen by all medical specialists. It is essential to identify them and either treat or refer appropriately.

Two basic abnormalities of mood are recognized: depression and mania. Both occur on a continuum from normal to the clearly pathologic—symptoms in a few patients reach psychotic proportions. Although minor symptoms may be an extension of normal sadness or elation, more severe symptoms are associated with discrete syndromes (mood disorders) that appear to differ qualitatively from normal processes and that require specific therapies.

CLASSIFICATION

DSM-IV has defined several different mood disorders that differ, among other things, in their clinical presentation, course, genetics, and treatment response. These conditions are distinguished from one another by (a) the presence or absence of mania (bipolar vs. unipolar), (b) the severity of the illness (major vs. minor), and (c) the role of medical or other psychiatric conditions in causing the disorder ($1°$ vs. $2°$):

I. **Major mood disorders:** *major* depressive and/or manic signs and symptoms.
   Bipolar I Disorder (manic-depression)—mania in past or present (with or without presence or history of depression). Major depression usually occurs sometime.

Bipolar II Disorder—*hypo*mania *and* major depression must be present or have been present sometime.

Major Depressive Disorder—serious depression alone.

II. **Other specific mood disorders:** *minor* depressive and/or manic signs and symptoms.

Dysthymic Disorder—depression alone.

Cyclothymic Disorder—depressive *and* hypomanic symptoms in the present or recent past (consistently over the past 2 years).

III. **Mood disorder due to a general medical condition** *and* **substance-induced mood disorder:** may be depressed, manic, or mixed; these are the 2° mood disorders.

IV. **Adjustment disorder with depressed mood:** depression caused by stress.

The DSM-IV classification also requires the examiner to specify whether the current bipolar episode is manic, depressed, or mixed; whether the unipolar or bipolar disorder is a single episode or recurrent and/or shows psychotic features, catatonia, rapid cycling, complete clearing between episodes, a seasonal pattern, or a postpartum onset; and whether a major depressive episode is *chronic* (present at least 2 years), meets the criteria for *melancholia* (profound vegetative and cognitive symptoms, including psychomotor retardation or agitation, sleep disturbance, anorexia or weight loss, and/or excessive guilt: see DSM-IV p. 384), or is *atypical* [increased appetite, weight gain, hypersomnia, interpersonal rejection sensitivity, "leaden" feeling in limbs: see DSM-IV p. 385 (1)]. These characteristics may be important in determining treatment and prognosis.

CLINICAL PRESENTATION OF MOOD DISORDERS

Of the core clinical features common to affective disturbances, the major mood disorders have the greater number and severity of symptoms and signs, whereas dysthymia and cyclothymia have fewer. The most common symptoms and signs of mood disorders are listed in Tables 4.1 and 4.2. A sufficient combination of these symptoms often clinches the diagnosis. However, particularly when the symptoms are mild, disorders of mood are frequently missed.

Although many depressed patients complain of depression, some do not. Moreover, other problems may obscure the diagnosis. Some patients present with alcohol or drug abuse or acting-out

TABLE 4.1 *Symptoms* **of Depression**

Emotional features
  Depressed mood, "blue"
  Irritability, anxiety
  Anhedonia, loss of interest
  Loss of zest
  Diminished emotional bonds
  Interpersonal withdrawal
  Preoccupation with death
Cognitive features
  Self-criticism, *sense of worthlessness,* guilt
  Pessimism, *hopelessness,* despair
  Distractible, *poor concentration*
  Uncertain and indecisive
  Variable obsessions
  Somatic complaints (*particularly in the elderly*)
  Memory impairment
  Delusions and hallucinations
Vegetative features
  Fatigability, no energy
  Insomnia or hypersomnia
  Anorexia or hyperrexia
  Weight loss or gain
  Psychomotor retardation
  Psychomotor agitation
  Impaired libido
  Frequent diurnal variation
Signs of depression
  Stooped and slow moving
  Tearful sad facies
  Dry mouth and skin
  Constipation

behavior. Others, particularly early on, present primarily with anxiety or agitation. Still others, instead of feeling sad, complain of *fatigue, insomnia,* dyspnea, tachycardia, and vague and/or chronic pains (usually GI, cardiac, headaches, or backaches—all unrelieved by analgesics) (2). People with such presentations (known as masked depression) often have a personal or family history of depression and frequently respond to antidepressants. Suspect depression in the unimproved patient who has atypical medical symptoms.

Patients with mania often do not complain of their symptoms. A few feel too good and elated to complain; others feel agitated

TABLE 4.2   *Symptoms* of Mania (When Nonpsychotic and Not Severe Enough to Impair Social or Occupational Functioning = Hypomania)

Emotional features
  Excited elevated mood, euphoria
  Emotional *lability*
  Rapid temporary shifts to acute depression
  Irritability, low frustration tolerance
  Demanding, egocentric
Cognitive features
  Elevated self-esteem, *grandiosity*
  Speech disturbances
  Loud word rhyming (clanging)
  Pressure of speech
  Flight of ideas
  Progression to incoherence
  Poor judgment, disorganization
  Paranoia
  Delusions and/or hallucinations
Physiologic features
  Boundless energy
  Insomnia, *little need for sleep*
  Decreased appetite
Signs of mania
  Psychomotor agitation

and unpleasant but fail to notice that their behavior is outrageous. Hypomanic patients can be irritable or "full of life," or both.

Patient rating scales can help determine the severity of a depression and can be used to measure change over time, e.g., the Beck Depression Inventory (21 questions—patient self-rates) and the Hamilton Rating Scale for Depression (17 to 21 questions—therapist rates).

NORMAL AFFECTIVE PROCESSES

Sadness or simple unhappiness affect us all from time to time. The cause is often obvious, the reaction understandable, and improvement follows the disappearance of the cause. However, prolonged unhappiness in response to a chronic stress may be indistinguishable from a minor affective disorder and require treatment. Support and improved life circumstances are the keys to recovery.

Grief or **BEREAVEMENT** (DSM-IV p. 684, V62.82) is a more profound sense of dysphoria that follows a severe loss or trauma and that may produce a full depressive syndrome but, as time distances the precipitating event, the symptoms disappear. This process often takes weeks or months and requires a "working through" that often includes disbelief, anger, intense mourning, and eventual resolution (see Chapter 10). Some bereavement grades into and, with time (e.g., longer than 2 months), becomes a major depressive disorder.

There is no generally accepted equivalent nonpathologic manic process, although some people do react to stress with hypomania.

MINOR AFFECTIVE DISORDERS

Depression

The common *chronic* nonpsychotic disorder of lowered mood and/or anhedonia is **DYSTHYMIC DISORDER** (DSM-IV p. 349, 300.4) (3). These patients feel depressed, have difficulty falling asleep, characteristically feel best in the morning and despondent in the afternoon and evening, and can display any of the nonpsychotic symptoms and signs of depression. Symptoms must have been present, at least intermittently, for 2 or more years. It is more common in women (F:M = 2–3:1), often develops for the first time in the late 20s or 30s, has a lifetime prevalence of 6%, and begins insidiously, frequently in a person predisposed to depression by

- Major loss in childhood (e.g., parent [maybe]);
- Recent loss (e.g., health, job, spouse);
- Chronic stress (e.g., medical disorder);
- Psychiatric susceptibility (e.g., personality disorders of histrionic, compulsive, and dependent types; alcohol and drug abuse; major depression in partial remission; obsessive-compulsive disorder—it frequently coexists with all these conditions).

It is similar to but less severe than a major depressive disorder; however, 20% or more of patients who experience major depression will clear incompletely and chronically suffer a residue of dysthymic disorder ("double depression"). It tends to last for many years.

Dysthymia must be differentiated from **ADJUSTMENT DISORDER WITH DEPRESSED MOOD** (DSM-IV p. 623, 309.0).

This disorder occurs in an adequately functioning individual shortly after a readily identifiable causative stress, results in impaired functioning, and resolves as the stress disappears. These patients present a depressive syndrome midway between normal sadness and major depression. If feelings of anxiety commingle with those of depression, the patient may have **ADJUSTMENT DISORDER WITH MIXED ANXIETY AND DEPRESSED MOOD** (DSM-IV p. 624, 309.28).

Hypomania

CYCLOTHYMIC DISORDER (DSM-IV p. 365, 301.13) requires the presence of mild depression *and* hypomania, separately or intermixed, continuously or intermittently over at least 2 years. It usually begins in the 20s in patients (F:M = 1:1) with a family history of major affective disorder and forms a chronically disabling pattern that yields troubled interpersonal relationships, job instability, occasional suicide attempts and short hospitalizations, and a markedly increased risk of drug and alcohol abuse.

MAJOR MOOD DISORDERS

Patients with major mood disorders are profoundly depressed or excited. Clinical presentations and genetic studies support two distinct groups, **MAJOR DEPRESSIVE DISORDER** (unipolar) (DSM-IV p. 344, 296.2x-.3x) and two types of bipolar disorders, **BIPOLAR I DISORDER** (DSM-IV p. 350, 296. xx) and **BIPOLAR II DISORDER** (DSM-IV p. 362, 296.89), yet some question this dichotomy (e.g., bipolar disorder *may* be a more severe form of recurrent unipolar disorder). The lifetime risk in the general population for a major depression is about 17% or more (4), ten times the frequency of bipolar disorder. Eventually, 15% of patients kill themselves.

Major Depression

These patients have many serious symptoms and signs of depression yet their clinical presentations can vary markedly—from profound retardation and withdrawal to irritable unrelieved agitation. A presumed precipitating event occurs in 25% (50% among the elderly) (5). A diurnal variation is common, with the most severe symptoms early in the day. Some fail to recognize their depression, complaining instead of their "insides rotting out" or their "minds going crazy," yet the profound affective disturbance is usually recognizable to the observer.

A thought disorder is occasionally present. Delusions are usually affect laden and mood congruent but need not be. Hallucinations are uncommon, auditory, and usually have a self-condemning or paranoid content. These "psychotic depressions" may represent a separate disorder or may simply be a more severe form of depression [mood disorder (M.D.) or bipolar disorder (B.D.) With Psychotic Features]. Depressed elderly may present primarily with retardation, memory impairment, and mild disorientation (*pseudodementia*).

The disorder can occur at any age (median age of onset is late 20s; 10% occur after age 60) with most cases spread evenly throughout the adult years and with females affected 2:1. (However, increasing numbers of teenagers and young adults seem to be afflicted.) Unlike schizophrenia, it occurs evenly in the higher social strata. Family and twin studies strongly suggest a genetic factor—increased incidence of major depression, alcoholism, and possibly antisocial personality disorder in relatives (the "depressive spectrum" disorders). The prevalence of serious affective illness in first-degree relatives is 13%, contrasted with 2%–4% in the general population. About 30%–40% of identical twins are concordant for unipolar depression. Alcoholism and chronic stress may predispose to the development of the illness. Molecular genetic "segregation and linkage analyses" has yet to identify a gene or chromosome for major depression despite strong (suggestive) evidence that this is a genetic illness.

Less than 50% of patients will have only one episode (M.D., Single Episode, 296.2x); 50%–60% have two or more attacks (M.D., Recurrent, 296.3x). Some patients clear between episodes, others remain mildly depressed (20%), and 10% are chronically severely depressed. Most attacks begin gradually over 1–3 weeks and, untreated, last from 3–8 months or longer. This is often a cyclic disorder: Relapse during the months or year or two after recovery from an acute episode is common (but partly avoidable with maintenance medication). These patients are often incapacitated during an episode and are at great risk of suicide. About half of the patients with recurrent illness will recover over 1–2 decades, whereas the rest will be chronically affected, although most will suffer dysthymia with infrequent relapses into major depression.

Postpartum depression is a severe depression usually beginning 1–2, and certainly by 4, weeks after delivery, usually of the second or third child. Affected women are at risk for repeated episodes with future deliveries.

Seasonal affective disorder (SAD) is characterized by the development of major depression with a seasonal pattern. Symptoms appear each fall/winter and return to normal (or even hypomania) during the spring/summer. It afflicts predominantly younger women (F:M = 2–4 : 1), displays many features of "atypical" depression (hypersomnia, weight gain, hyperphagia), and is often treated successfully with bright artificial light (2–6 hr/day with a response in 2–3 days; occasionally, hypomania occurs) with or without antidepressants (6). Its relationship to more classic major depression is unclear.

The apparent biologic nature of many serious depressions is reflected in the recent development of several putative biologic tests for depression:

- *Dexamethasone suppression test* (DST) (positive test is the failure of normal suppression of plasma cortisol 6–24 hours after an oral dose of dexamethasone);
- *Elevated serum cortisol* (30% of patients have adrenal hypertrophy);
- *Decreased urinary MHPG* (3-methoxy-4-hydroxyphenyleneglycol, a catabolite of norepinephrine) and CSF 5-HIAA (a metabolite of serotonin);
- *TRH stimulation test* (low TSH and blunted TSH and GH responses to exogenous TRH suggest unipolar depression);
- Sleep abnormalities: *short REM latency*—time from falling asleep to start of REM sleep (a *very* good indicator); *frequent awakenings; early morning awakenings;* decreased NREM sleep; *increased REM density* (frequency of rapid eye movements in REM sleep). These all may be traits in people prone to depression;
- *Stimulant challenge tests* (some depressed patients briefly improve when given 10 mg of amphetamine).

Unfortunately, these tests have little routine clinical utility; the best seem to be (a) abnormal sleep studies, (b) abnormal

TSH levels and TRH responses, and (c) a *posttreatment* positive DST as a measure of poor outcome. These tests all suffer from inadequate sensitivity and specificity (too many false positives and negatives). However, each further emphasizes that biology plays a role in many depressions. (Still, environment also plays a role because 25% of patients with serious medical conditions and others suffering marked psychosocial stress will develop a major depression.)

Searching for the CNS site(s) of the illness with PET and fMRI has been more promising, suggesting that major depression is associated (somehow) with decreased activity in the lateral prefrontal cortex (particularly the left side), the caudate, the putamen, and probably also the amygdala (7,8).

Bipolar Disorders

Mania, at some time severe enough to produce compromised functioning, is necessary to diagnose **bipolar I disorder,** but 90% or more of patients also have periods of depression (B.D., Depressed, 296. 5x). The manic episode typically develops over days and may become uncontrolled and psychotic (B.D., Manic, 296.4x). About 20% or more of manics have hallucinations and/or delusions. A severe mania may be indistinguishable from an organic delirium (sudden onset, anorexia, insomnia, disorientation, paranoia, hallucinations, and delusions) or acute schizophrenia. When the bipolar patient is depressed, the depression is *usually* profound but occasionally may present as a mild depressive syndrome. Attacks usually are separated by months or years, but the patient occasionally may cycle from one to the other over days or weeks [*With Rapid Cycling* (DSM-IV p. 391)—four or more mood episodes in a year; 10% or more of patients; F:M = 4:1; younger; poorer prognosis; but the pattern may disappear] or actually present contrasting symptoms simultaneously (e.g., spirited singing intermixed with crying; B.D., Mixed, 296.6x). This is a recurrent illness—single attacks are rare. Pure manic syndromes (patients who have only mania—*unipolar mania*) occur clinically but are unusual and are probably not a separate entity.

Bipolar II disorder occurs when a patient who has had a major depression also experiences a hypomanic episode (usually around the time of the depression) but never gets fully manic. It occurs more frequently in women who have a family history of mood disorder; 10% or more go on to develop bipolar I disorder by later having a manic episode.

The lifetime risk for developing bipolar disorder is approximately 1.0%[+]. This is a genetic disorder. First-degree relatives are at risk for bipolar disorder (5%–10% develop it), major depression (10%[+]), and cyclothymia. There is a 70% or more concordance for bipolar illness in identical twins. In contrast with major depression, M:F = 1:1. The type of inheritance is uncertain but is almost certainly genetically heterogeneous and polygenic. Countless linkage studies suggest at least a dozen different chromosomes and even more different locations (9).

The first manic episode is often before age 30, begins quickly, and resolves in 2–4 months if untreated. One or more episodes of depression usually have already occurred. Most patients go on to have a majority of depressive episodes. Suicide is the major risk (almost 20% lifetime risk) during periods of depression. Legal difficulties and drug and alcohol abuse (as well as suicide) occur with manic periods.

MOOD DISORDER DUE TO A GENERAL MEDICAL CONDITION

Various medical conditions can directly produce major depressive and/or manic syndromes (DSM-IV p. 369, 293.83), although who will develop such a syndrome is unpredictable. Some illnesses have a high likelihood of producing a mood disturbance (e.g., depression in 50% or more of patients with stroke, pancreatic carcinoma, and Cushing's syndrome), whereas it is much less common, but no less direct, with other illnesses. This disorder is *not* meant for those medical conditions that produce depression or mania as a reaction to having the illness nor for those patients who only show a mood disturbance when delirious. Likely medical diseases include (see Chapters 14 and 15)

- **Depression**
  Tumors—particularly of *brain* and *lung, carcinoma of pancreas* (50% develop psychiatric symptoms *before* the diagnosis is made)
  Infections—*influenza,* mononucleosis, "flu-fatigue" syndrome (EB virus?), encephalitis, hepatitis

Endocrine disorders—Cushing's disease (60% of patients; also from exogenous steroids), *hypothyroidism* (some experts recommend a careful thyroid evaluation in most (all?) depressed patients), apathetic hyperthyroidism, hyperparathyroidism (symptoms parallel levels of serum Ca^{2+}), diabetes, Turner's syndrome

Blood—anemia (particularly pernicious anemia)

Nutrition and electrolytes—pellagra, hyponatremia, hypokalemia, hypercalcemia, inappropriate ADH

Miscellaneous—MS, *Parkinson's disease,* head trauma, *stroke* [poststroke depression, particularly L-frontal (?)], early Huntington's disease, *MI,* premenstrual syndrome (?), menopause (relieved by estrogens)

- **Mania**

  Tumors—of brain

  Infections—encephalitis, influenza, syphilis (20% of patients with general paresis)

  Miscellaneous—MS, Wilson's disease, head trauma, psychomotor epilepsy, hyperthyroidism

SUBSTANCE-INDUCED MOOD DISORDER

Drugs of abuse, medications, and toxins all can produce mood disorders of various types (DSM-IV p. 374). The likelihood of mood symptoms from use of a substance and the pattern of symptoms produced varies not only with the specific drug but also with the dose, the duration of use, whether the issue is intoxication or withdrawal, and ill-specified and poorly understood individual factors in the patient. A modest list of likely agents include (see Chapter 13)

- **Depression**

  Drugs of abuse—alcohol (often hard to tell "which is the chicken and which the egg"), sedative-hypnotics, opioids, PCP

  Medication—oral contraceptives, *corticosteroids, reserpine* (6% of patients), *alpha-methyldopa,* guanethidine, *levodopa, indomethacin,* benzodiazepines, opiates, *cimetidine, propranolol,* anticholinesterases, amphetamine withdrawal

  Miscellaneous—heavy metal poisoning

- **Mania**

  Drugs of abuse—cocaine, amphetamines, hallucinogens, PCP

Medication—steroids, L-dopa
Miscellaneous—organophosphates, petroleum distillates

MOOD DISORDER NOS

BIPOLAR DISORDER NOS (DSM-IV p. 366, 296.80) and **DEPRESSIVE DISORDER NOS** (DSM-IV p. 350, 311) include the remaining (unusual) affective presentations.

DIFFERENTIAL DIAGNOSIS

Depression

- **Schizophrenic Disorders:** Particularly catatonics, but any type can look or be depressed during or after an episode. Poor premorbid adjustment, formal thought disorder with well-formed delusions and complex hallucinations, lack of cyclic history, and no family history for affective disorder all suggest schizophrenia.
- **Schizoaffective Disorder:** A psychotic disorder that meets the criteria for schizophrenia but with superimposed major mood symptoms for part of the time.
- **Generalized Anxiety Disorder:** Anxiety appears first and predominates. With the anxious patient, *always* consider depression.
- **Alcoholism and Drug Abuse:** Alcoholism and depression are both often present ("dual diagnosis" patients).
- **Obsessive-Compulsive Disorder, Histrionic and Borderline Personality Disorders:** Are the full syndromes present?
- **Dementia:** "Pseudodepression" is common and differentiation is tricky, particularly in the elderly. Check for memory impairment and disorientation.

Mania

- **Schizophrenic Disorders:** Often indistinguishable in acute cases. Check past personal and family history.
- **Schizoaffective Disorder**
- **Borderline Personality Disorder**

PSYCHOBIOLOGIC THEORIES

Psychoanalytic theory (Freud) postulates that a depressed patient has suffered a real or imagined loss of an ambivalently loved object, has reacted with unconscious rage that has been then turned against the self, and this has resulted in a lowered self-esteem and depression. *Cognitive theory* postulates a "cognitive triad" of distorted perceptions in which (a) a person's negative interpretation of his or her own life experiences (b) causes a devaluation of him or herself that (c) causes depression.

Promising but unproven *biologic* theories focus on brain nor-epinephrine (NE) and serotonin (5-HT) abnormalities. Biologic and psychological theories need not be mutually exclusive. The *catecholamine hypothesis* suggests that low brain NE levels cause depression and elevated levels cause mania; however, urinary MHPG levels (a major metabolite of NE) are low in only some depressions. The *indolamine hypothesis* holds that low cerebral 5-HT (or the primary metabolite, 5-HIAA) causes depression and elevation causes mania, yet exceptions occur. The *permissive hypothesis* postulates that lowered NE produces depression and raised NE causes mania only if 5-HT levels are low. The known mechanisms of action of antidepressants support these theories—tricyclics block NE and 5-HT reuptake and monoamine oxidase inhibitors block oxidation of NE. In addition, recent research suggests that there may be frontal lobe/whole brain hypometabolism in depression or some fundamental abnormality of the circadian rhythms of depressed patients.

TREATMENT OF DEPRESSION

Evaluate medically and psychiatrically to rule out secondary depression and to attempt to identify an affective syndrome. Always ask about vegetative features and evaluate suicidal potential (see Chapter 7). If the patient (a) is incapacitated by the disorder, (b) has a destructive home environment or limited environmental support, (c) is a suicide risk, or (d) has an associated medical illness requiring treatment, hospitalize. All depressed patients should receive psychotherapy; some must receive physical therapies in addition. The specific treatments used depend on the diagnosis, severity, patient age, and past responses to therapy.

Psychological Therapies

Supportive psychotherapy is always indicated. Be warm, empathic, understanding, and optimistic. Help the patient to identify and express concerns and to ventilate. Identify precipitating factors and help correct. Help solve external problems (e.g., rent, job)—be directive, particularly during the acute episode and if the patient is immobilized. Train the patient to recognize signs of future decompensation. See the patient frequently (1–3 times/week initially) and regularly but not interminably—be available. Recognize that some depressed patients can provoke anger in you (via anger, hostility, unreasonable demands, etc.)—watch for it. Long-term *insight-oriented psychotherapy* may be of value in selected chronic minor depressions and some conflicted patients with a major depression in remission.

   Cognitive-behavior therapy is very useful with mild to moderately severe depressives (10). Believed by some to be "learned helplessness," depressions are treated by giving patients skill training and providing success experiences. From a cognitive perspective, the patient is trained to recognize and eliminate negative thoughts and expectations. This therapy helps prevent relapse (11,12).

   Partial sleep deprivation (awaken midway through the night and keep up until the next evening) helps lessen the symptoms of a major depression temporarily. Physical exercise (running, swimming) may produce improvement in depression, for poorly understood biologic reasons.

Physical Therapies (see Chapter 23)

All major and most chronic or unimproved minor depressions require a trial of antidepressants (70%–80% of patients respond), even though an apparent precipitant of the depression is identified. Begin with an SSRI or one of the newer antidepressants. If that fails, consider a *tricyclic* antidepressant, an *MAOI* (particularly in "atypical" depressions), or one of numerous effective drug combinations if the first drug fails. Be alert to side effects and be aware that antidepressants "may" precipitate a manic episode in a few bipolar patients (10% with TCAs; possibly lower with SSRI—but recognize that the whole "manic precipitation" concept is debated). Maintain for several months after remission from a first depressive episode and then taper; however, many patients, after one or more relapses, will require maintenance medication for long periods (13). An antidepressant rarely is sufficient alone in treating a unipolar psychotic depression.

Lithium is effective at producing a remission in bipolar disorders, mania, and it *may* be useful in treating acute bipolar depressions and a few unipolar depressions. It is moderately effective at maintaining a remission in bipolar and some unipolar patients as well. *Anticonvulsants* seem to be at least as good as lithium at treating the acute conditions, although perhaps less effective at maintenance (14). Antidepressants and lithium may be started concurrently, and the lithium continued after remission. Psychotic, paranoid, or very agitated patients may require an *antipsychotic,* alone or with an antidepressant, lithium, or ECT— the new atypical antipsychotics seem particularly effective.

ECT may be the treatment of choice (a) if medication fails after one or more 6-week trials, (b) if the patient's condition demands an immediate remission (e.g., *acutely* suicidal), (c) in some psychotic depressions, or (d) in patients who cannot tolerate medication (e.g., some elderly cardiac patients). Up to 90% of patients respond.

TREATMENT OF MANIA

Evaluate carefully but quickly. Is the patient medically ill or taking drugs? Has he or she been manic before? Is he or she taking lithium? What is the blood level?

If hypomanic, use outpatient treatment and work with the family, if possible. Consider short-term low-dose antipsychotics (e.g., haloperidol 2–5 mg/day) but rely on treatment with lithium or anticonvulsants longer term. *If manic,* hospitalize. Is the patient debilitated? Seriously sleep deprived?

1. Medicate acutely with antipsychotics (large doses may be required, e.g., haloperidol 10–40 mg, during the first 24 hours). Consider adjunctive use of a benzodiazepine early on. Also, if drugs fail, ECT is an effective treatment for acute mania.
2. Be relaxed, reasonable, and controlled. Treat in quiet setting with minimal stimuli. Set firm limits.
3. Begin lithium carbonate; however, as many as 30% of manics stay partially symptomatic despite lithium. If lithium fails, consider *carbamazepine, valproic acid,* or one of the other anticonvulsants. Even with proper treatment, long-term outcome is often poor.

REFERENCES

1. Nierenberg AA, Alpert JE, Pava J, et al. Course and treatment of atypical depression. *J Clin Psychiatry* 1998;59[Suppl 18]:5–9.
2. Posse M, Hällström. Depressive disorders among somatizing patients in primary health care. *Acta Psychiatr Scand* 1998;98:187–192.
3. Klein DN, Norden KA, Ferro T, et al. Thirty-month naturalistic follow-up study of early-onset dysthymic disorder. *J Abnorm Psychol* 1998;107: 338–348.
4. Blazer DG, Kessler RC, McGonagle KA, et al. The prevalence and distribution of major depression in a national community sample: the National Comorbidity Survey. *Am J Psychiatry* 1994;151:979–986.
5. Cui X, Vaillant GE. Antecedents and consequences of negative life events in adulthood. *Am J Psychiatry* 1996;152:21–26.
6. Lewy AJ, Bauer VK, Cutler NL, et al. Morning vs. evening light treatment of patients with winter depression. *Arch Gen Psychiatry* 1998;55: 890–896.
7. Kennedy SH, Javanmard M, Vaccarino FJ. A review of functional neuroimaging in mood disorders: positron emission tomography and depression. *Can J Psychiatry* 1997;42:467–475.
8. Soares JC, Mann JJ. The anatomy of mood disorders—review of structural neuroimaging studies. *Biol Psychiatry* 1997;41:86–106.
9. Gershon ES, Badner JA, Goldin LR, et al. Closing in on genes for manic-depressive illness and schizophrenia. *Neuropsychopharmacology* 1998;18:233–242.
10. Jørgensen MB, Dam H, Bolwig TG. The efficacy of psychotherapy in non-bipolar depression: a review. *Acta Psychiatr Scand* 1998;98:1–13.
11. DeRubeis RJ, Gelfand LA, Tang TZ, et al. Medications versus cognitive behavior therapy for severely depressed outpatients: mega-analysis of four randomized comparisons. *Am J Psychiatry* 1999;156:1007–1013.
12. Fava GA, Rafanelli C, Grandi S, et al. Prevention of recurrent depression with cognitive behavioral therapy. *Arch Gen Psychiatry* 1998;55: 816–820.
13. Mueller TI, Leon AC, Keller MB, et al. Recurrence after recovery from major depressive disorder during 15 years of observational follow-up. *Am J Psychiatry* 1999;156:1000–1006.
14. Gadde KM, Krishnan KRR. Recent advances in the pharmacologic treatment of bipolar illness. *Psychiatric Ann* 1997;27:496–506.

Chapter 5

Delirium and Amnestic and Other Cognitive Disorders

The psychiatric conditions in this chapter are all caused by medical (organic) pathology. The most common is delirium, but several other specific presentations occur as well. In addition, organic processes contribute to dementia (see Chapter 6), intoxication and withdrawal (see Chapters 16 and 17), and many of the syndromes found in other chapters.

These syndromes are common, particularly among the elderly (20% or more of all acute medical inpatients develop some organic syndrome, usually delirium). Delirium is usually brief and reversible, and dementia is longer lasting and more likely to be irreversible, yet none of these characterizations is completely true (e.g., 15%–20% of dementias are reversible). These conditions are clinically defined, and their course and characteristics depend on the nature, severity, course, and location of the causative organic pathology. First, identify the syndrome, and then determine the likely organic cause.

DELIRIUM

Delirium (1) is a common condition that may be caused by physical illness (**D. DUE TO A GENERAL MEDICAL CONDITION,** DSM-IV p. 129, 293.0), drugs (**SUBSTANCE INTOXICATION OR WITHDRAWAL D.,** DSM-IV p. 131), several causes simultaneously (**D. DUE TO MULTIPLE ETIOLOGIES,** DSM-IV p. 132), or by unknown organic conditions. These patients may be confused, bizarre, or even "wild" and thus can be mistakenly thought to be suffering from other psychotic illnesses. Other delirious patients may appear somnolent or perfectly normal during the day but decompensate dramatically in the evening or night. Still other patients may have increasing difficulty functioning due to a mild delirium that is only revealed by specific mental status testing (2). Synonyms include acute brain syndrome, toxic psychosis, acute confusional state, and metabolic encephalopathy.

Diagnosis

Delirium is a rapidly developing disorder of disturbed attention that fluctuates with time. Although the clinical presentation of delirium differs considerably from patient to patient, there are several characteristic features that help to make the diagnosis:

- **Clouding of consciousness:** The patient is not normally alert and may appear bewildered and confused. There may be noticeably decreased alertness (grading into stupor) or hyperalertness. Observe the patient.
- **Attention deficit:** The patient usually is very distractible and unable to focus attention sufficiently or for a long enough time to follow a train of thought or to understand what is occurring around him. Have the patient do serial 7's and/or a Random Letter Test.
- **Perceptual disturbances:** These are common and include misinterpretations of environmental events, illusions (e.g., the curtain blows and the patient believes someone is climbing in the window), and hallucinations (usually visual). The patient may or may not recognize these misperceptions as unreal.
- **Sleep–wake alteration:** Insomnia is almost always present (all symptoms are usually worse at night and in the dark) and marked drowsiness may also occur.
- **Disorientation:** Most frequently to time but also to place, situation, and (finally) person. Ask for the date, time, and day of the week: "What place is this?," etc.
- **Memory impairment:** The patient typically has a recent memory deficit and usually denies it (he or she may confabulate and may want to talk about the distant past). Ask about the recent past, e.g., "Who brought you to the hospital?" "Did you have any tests yesterday?" "What did you have for breakfast?," etc. Name four objects and two words and ask the patient for them in 5 minutes. Does he or she remember your name?

- **Incoherence:** The patient may attempt to communicate but the speech may be confused or even unintelligible. Verbal perseveration may occur.
- **Altered psychomotor activity:** Most delirious patients are restless and agitated and may display perseveration of motion, some may be excessively somnolent, and some may fluctuate from one to the other (usually restless at night and sleepy during the day).
- **Fluctuations:** Most of the characteristics listed above vary in severity *over hours* and days.

A delirium usually develops over days and *may* precede signs of the organic condition causing it. Usually it lasts less than a week (depending on the cause). Many of these patients are significantly anxious or frightened by their experiences, may become combative, and may develop some delusional ideas based on their misperceptions. A few patients become dangerously suicidal—watch for it. Environmental conditions can significantly alter the presentation of a delirium. Change of setting (e.g., moving out of familiar surroundings), overstimulation, and understimulation (e.g., darkness, sensory deprivation) can all worsen the symptoms, as can stress of any kind.

It is necessary to have a high index of suspicion and to ask specific mental status questions if you are going to identify delirium early. Ask questions tactfully because many patients defensively resist this probing. The early prodromal symptoms that should alert you to a developing delirium include

Restlessness (particularly at night), anxiety;
Daytime somnolence;
Insomnia, vivid dreams, and nightmares;
Hypersensitivity to light and sound;
Fleeting illusions and hallucinations;
Distractibility, difficulty in thinking clearly.

The EEG (although usually not necessary to make the diagnosis) has a characteristic pattern of *diffuse slowing* that is proportional to the severity of the delirium. It can help if there is a question of the presence of a functional psychosis, drug use, or a dissociative state. Delirium may also be accompanied by a tremor, asterixis, diaphoresis, tachycardia, elevated BP, tachypnea, and flushing.

Etiology and Differential Diagnosis

The presence of a delirium usually means that the patient is seriously medically ill (3). Delirium is a diagnosis that demands an immediate search for causes. Most causes produce diffuse cerebral impairment and lie *outside* the CNS—usually due to some form of deranged metabolism (e.g., infection, fever, hypoxia, hypoglycemia, medication side effects, drug withdrawal states, hepatic encephalopathy, postoperative changes)—but also include CNS trauma and postictal states. The specific potential etiologies are too numerous to list (consult a more complete source), although usually the cause is evident. These patients all deserve a thorough physical and laboratory examination.

The major problem in differential diagnosis is in distinguishing a delirium from a psychotic disorder. The delirious patient is usually more acute and confused, and the hallucinations are usually more disorganized and are more likely to be visual. Typical psychotic disorders usually do not have confusion, disorientation, and illusions, and they are more likely to have a formal thought disorder. *Always* check the personal and family history for serious psychiatric illness.

Treatment

The following are guidelines in treating delirium (4):

- Provide adequate medical care for an identified cause of the delirium. Patients with delirium have an increased mortality rate.
- Provide for the patient's safety. Maintain around-the-clock observation (particularly at night). This may require someone in the room constantly—preferably someone with whom the patient is familiar. Use restraints only if absolutely necessary (they frequently increase agitation).
- Keep the patient in a quiet well-lighted room. Keep familiar objects around and use the same treatment personnel, if possible.
- Frequently (and tactfully) reorient the patient. Introduce yourself again and describe what you are doing and why.
- Anticipate the patient's anxiety and reassure him. Be calm and sympathetic.
- Medication should be used cautiously. Use low doses. If psychotic features are prevalent, consider haloperidol or chlor-

promazine (5). If sedation is called for (usually for marked agitation), consider the benzodiazepines (e.g., diazepam, clonazepam).

The following organic syndromes are considerably less common than delirium, dementia, and the substance abuse syndromes of intoxication and withdrawal. They are also more likely to be associated with focal organic pathology and with a few specific medical or neurologic diseases.

AMNESTIC SYNDROME (DUE TO A GENERAL MEDICAL CONDITION; DSM-IV p. 160, 294.0) (SUBSTANCE-INDUCED; DSM-IV p. 162)

These patients have severe memory deficits that usually appear suddenly after a CNS insult and that may become chronic. The deficits are *both* retrograde (old memories—ask about childhood, schooling, etc.) and anterograde (new memory—ask the patient to remember several facts for 5–10 minutes). The patients are often unaware that their memory is impaired. Unlike delirium, the sensorium is usually clear, although there may be disorientation. Unlike dementia, serious memory loss occurs without intellectual or other associated changes.

There are numerous potential causes that include CNS trauma, hypoxia, herpes simplex encephalitis, and some substance abuse (particularly alcohol and sedative-hypnotic abuse) (see Chapters 16 and 17). Bilateral lesions of the medial temporal and/or diencephalic regions appear to be required. Treatment consists of correcting any medical/organic causes; and waiting.

CATATONIC DISORDER DUE TO A GENERAL MEDICAL CONDITION (DSM-IV p. 170, 393.89)

These patients display *catatonia* (immobility—stuporousness or the "waxy flexibility" of catalepsy—but sometimes extreme agitation; also mutism, slow and stereotyped movements, echolalia, and/or echopraxia) caused by a medical condition or a substance. The most common causes are neurologic and metabolic (e.g., hypercalcemia or hepatic encephalopathy). Be sure to rule out catatonic schizophrenia (history of psychosis; no medical causes) but do not assume every catatonic patient is "just schizophrenic."

PERSONALITY CHANGE DUE TO A GENERAL MEDICAL CONDITION (DSM-IV p. 173, 310.1)

These patients display a personality *change* or a marked exacerbation of previous personality characteristics. Often this takes the form of a loss of control over impulses and emotions or the development of apathy, irritability, aggression, paranoia, or indifference. Impairment of social judgment is common. The usual cause is frontal lobe damage (the frontal lobe syndrome) due to stroke, tumor, CNS trauma, normal pressure hydrocephalus, general paresis, Huntington's chorea, or MS. Occasionally, right-sided strokes may be responsible. Be careful not to mistake it for mild delirium or the early changes of dementia, schizophrenia, or major affective disorder.

REFERENCES

1. Lipowski ZJ. *Delirium.* New York: Oxford University Press, 1990.
2. Hill CD, Risby E, Morgan N. Cognitive deficits in delirium: assessment over time. *Psychopharmacol Bull* 1992;28:401–407.
3. Weddington WW. The mortality of delirium: an underappreciated problem? *Psychosomatics* 1982;23:1232–1234.
4. Work Group on Delirium. Practice guideline for the treatment of patients with delirium. *Am J Psychiatry* 1999;156[Suppl 5]:1–20.
5. Breitbart W, Marotta R, Platt MM, et al. A double-blind trial of haloperidol, chlorpromazine, and lorazepam in the treatment of delirium in hospitalized AIDS patients. *Am J Psychiatry* 1996;153: 231–237.

Chapter 6

Dementia

DEMENTIA (DSM-IV p. 133) results from a broad loss of intellectual functions due to diffuse organic disease of (a) the cerebral hemispheres (*cortical dementia*) or the (b) subcortical structures (*subcortical dementia*, e.g., Huntington's and Parkinson's diseases) of sufficient severity to impair social and/or occupational functioning. Dementia is a clinical presentation demanding a diagnosis—*not* a diagnosis itself. Causes are numerous, but clinical presentations are remarkably similar. Sixty percent of dementias are irreversible, but because 25% are controllable and 15% are reversible, treatable causes must be identified.

MAKING THE DIAGNOSIS

Dementia usually develops slowly and is easily overlooked. A rapid onset suggests a recent (and possibly treatable) insult, although frequently a mild unrecognized dementia is made worse and obvious by a medical illness (e.g., pneumonia, CHF). *Always* interview the family—they frequently notice changes (in personality, memory, etc.) of which the patient is unaware. Unlike delirium, clouding of consciousness is minimal (unless dementia and delirium are mixed)—make sure the patient is alert (1).

EARLY—Effects include subtle changes in personality, impaired social skills, a decrease in the range of interests and enthusiasms, lability and shallowness of affect, agitation, numerous somatic complaints, vague psychiatric symptoms, and a gradual loss of intellectual skills and acuity. These are often first noticed in work settings where high performance is required. Patients may recognize a loss of abilities initially but vigorously deny it. Early dementia often precipitates a depression. Remember: early dementia may present primarily with emotional (usually depressive) rather than cognitive symptoms, *but also* emotional disorders may mimic early dementia. Do not under- or overdiagnose it.

LATE—Parts of the full picture emerge:

- **Memory loss:** Usually immediate and recent memory loss [hippocampus (2)] but gradually involves remote recall (medial temporal and diencephalic regions involved). Does the patient forget appointments, the news, people he or she has just met, or places he or she has just been? Patient may confabulate, so check the information. Ask the patient to (a) repeat digits (normal, remember 6 forward, 4 backward) and (b) recall 2 words and 3 objects after 5 minutes. Does the patient know your name? the nurse? this place? the names of his or her visitors? last night's meal? Does the patient know his or her birth date? hometown? the name of his or her high school?

- **Changes in mood and personality:** Often exaggeration of previous personality (e.g., more compulsive or more excitable). *Depression,* anxiety, and/or irritability early on—later, withdrawal and apathy. Has the patient become sloppy, belligerent, thoughtless of others, *paranoid,* socially inappropriate, fearful? Does he lack initiative or interest? Use vulgar language or jokes?

- **Loss of orientation:** Particularly time (of day, day of week, date, season) but also place ("What place is this?") and, when severe, person. Has the patient been getting lost—in new places? in the former neighborhood? at home? Does the patient know why he or she is here (situation)? The patient may not sleep well, wander around at night, and get lost.

- **Intellectual impairment:** Patient is "less sharp" than he or she used to be. Does the patient have trouble doing things he or she could previously do easily? General information (last 5 presidents, 6 large U.S. cities), calculations (multiplication tables, serial 7's, make change), similarities (how are a ball and an orange alike? a mouse and an elephant? a fly and a tree?).

- **Compromised judgment:** Does not anticipate consequences. Does the patient act impulsively? "What should you do if you found a stamped addressed envelope?" "If you noticed a fire in a theater?"

- **Psychotic symptoms:** Hallucinations (usually simple), illusions, delusions, unshakable preoccupations, ideas of reference.
- **Language impairment:** Often vague and imprecise; occasionally almost mute. Is there perseveration, blocking, or aphasia? (With early aphasia, suspect focal pathology.)

Ask about history of chronic medical or psychiatric disease, family psychiatric illness, drug or alcohol abuse, head injury, and exposure to toxins.

Physical Examination

Examine for the numerous medical causes of dementia—e.g., endocrine, heart, kidney, lung, liver, infection (see below). Always perform a careful neurologic examination and identify any focal CNS causes of dementia. Always test for sense of smell (1st cranial nerve)—may identify a large unrecognized frontal lobe lesion. Always test hearing. Advanced diffuse disease displays ataxia, facial grimaces, agnosias, apraxias, motor impersistence, and/or perseveration and pathologic reflexes (grasp, snout, suck, glabella tap, tonic foot, etc.). Recognize that all types of physical illnesses occur more frequently in the demented patient (reasons for this are unclear). Survival time is reduced.

Laboratory Examination

Select tests based on suspected etiology. Consider screening with ESR, CBC, STS, SMA-12, T_3 & T_4, vitamin B_{12} and folate assays, UA, chest x-ray, and CT scan. Other tests based on likely causes include drug levels, EEG (20% of all elderly have an abnormal EEG), LP (rarely), arteriography, etc. The EEG is useful for identifying pathology in the usually silent CNS areas (frontal and temporal lobes)—investigate further if the dementia is mild but the EEG is grossly abnormal.

Psychological Testing

These can (a) help identify a focal lesion, (b) provide a baseline, (c) help with the diagnosis, and (d) identify strengths to be used in planning treatment. Useful tests include the WAIS, Bender-Gestalt Test, the Luria test, and the Halstead and Reitan Batteries (very time consuming; do not use routinely). A brief but useful screening test is the Mini-Mental State Exam (3). Patients with even mild dementia often will show impaired *constructional ability;* thus, have them draw simple figures (e.g., a diamond, a cross, and a cube or the face of a clock set at a certain time—can be done on initial interview). Repeat drawings can be used to track the illness over time (4).

CAUSES

Major Untreatable Dementias

DEMENTIA OF THE ALZHEIMER TYPE (AD) (DSM-IV p. 142, 290.xx)

Approximately 50%+ of all dementias (5%–10% of people over 65; 50% over 85) but usually a diagnosis by exclusion. AD (5) is the "classic cortical dementia." It is frequently overdiagnosed. Typically begins insidiously in the 50s (early onset, familial, presenile form—2% of cases) or later in the 60s to 80s (much more common late-onset form) and progresses to death in 6–10 years (6). Ceaseless pacing and a shuffling gait are common; social responses often remain intact until very late. Look for cortical atrophy and enlarged ventricles by MRI. The EEG is often normal for age early on but is a good screening test because it is often abnormal with reversible causes of dementia (except for general paresis and NPH). Histologically, there are senile plaques (degenerated nerve terminals surrounding a neurotoxic β-amyloid core), neurofibrillary tangles, and neuronal granulovacuolar degeneration. Recent evidence implicates primary degeneration of cholinergic neurons of the basal forebrain, particularly the nucleus basalis (although serotonergic and other neurons are increasingly being implicated—very heterogeneous).

There is an increased incidence in women (1.5:1), first-degree relatives threefold, particularly with presenile dementia), and Down's syndrome. [Moreover, a few early onset familial cases have been related to the amyloid precursor protein gene (*APP* gene; increased production and/or deposition of amyloid β-protein over years or decades) on the portion of chromosome 21 near the region associated with Down's syndrome. Other cases have been associated with chromosome 14 (presenilin 1 gene) and a third group with the presenilin 2 gene on chromosome 1. On the other hand, "normal" (98% of cases) late-onset AD has been associated with the apolipoprotein E type 4 (apoE ε4) allele on chromosome

19 (7) and recently with the *A2M* gene on chromosome 12. Clearly, other genes are yet to be found for late-onset AD.]

Huntington's Chorea   This is a subcortical dementia. Psychiatric symptoms, ranging from neurotic to psychotic (including dementia), may precede the chorea. Dementia always occurs terminally. This disease is autosomal dominant (short arm of chromosome 4) so check family history.

Parkinson's Disease   Lesion in the basal ganglia (subcortical). Depression (40%) and/or dementia in some patients. Levodopa relieves temporarily only.

Others   Other causes include progressive supranuclear palsy, spinocerebellar degenerations, Pick's disease, parkinsonism–dementia complex of Guam, SSPE, Creutzfeldt-Jakob disease, herpes simplex encephalitis, MS, HIV, and head trauma.

Treatable Forms of Dementia

VASCULAR DEMENTIA (DSM-IV p. 146, 290.4x)
These are 10% of dementias. Differentiate from AD by history of rapid onset and stepwise deterioration (can be difficult) in a patient in his 50s or early 60s and by presence of focal neurologic impairment. EEG may show focal abnormalities. Caused by multiple thromboembolic episodes (numerous small cerebral infarcts pathologically) in a patient with atherosclerotic disease of the major vessels or valvular disease of the heart. Hypertension is usually present. Pseudobulbar phenomena are common: emotional lability, dysarthria, and dysphagia. Controlling BP may help slow progression.

Normal Pressure Hydrocephalus (NPH)   A "classic triad" of *gait ataxia, incontinence,* and *progressive dementia*—either idiopathic or after cerebral trauma, hemorrhage, or infection. There is normal CSF pressure but dilated ventricles by MRI. Treat with a lumboperitoneal or ventriculoatrial shunt; 55% show improvement.

SUBSTANCE-INDUCED PERSISTING DEMENTIA (DSM-IV p. 154)
A diagnosis by exclusion. Most commonly follows many years of heavy drinking and may be partly reversible with good nutrition

and abstinence. Also, secondary to chronic sedative-hypnotic abuse and toxins like lead, mercury, solvents, and organophosphates. Possible causes include

- **Drug intoxication:** Common, particularly in the elderly (too many medications, misunderstood instructions, etc.). Watch for major and minor tranquilizers, analgesics (particularly phenacetin), digoxin, primidone, phenacemide, methyldopa. Reevaluate and stop, if possible.
- **Brain tumors:** Primarily metastatic tumors (from lung and breast) and meningiomas. Focal signs are usually present except in frontal lobe. Get CSF pressure and protein, EEG, and MRI. EEG may be localizing.
- **Brain trauma:** Dementia is unusual except for *subdural hematoma* in the elderly—dementia, headache, and drowsiness developing over weeks or months with or without a history of trauma. Do not do an LP. Get CT or MRI, then arteriography (diagnostic). *May* be reversible.
- **Infection:** Any significant infection (e.g., pneumonia, UTI) can produce delirium and worsen a dementia in the elderly. Dementia can be caused by brain abscess, CNS syphilis (general paresis - serologic tests of blood and CSF usually positive), and tuberculosis and cryptococcal meningitis.
- **Metabolic disorders:** Most common are thyroid disorders—*hypothyroidism* (dementia even with near-normal hormone levels; may be reversible; look for diffuse slowing on EEG) and also hyperthyroidism ("apathetic thyrotoxicosis," particularly in the elderly). Electrolyte imbalances are also common causes in the elderly, e.g., hypo- and hypernatremia and hypercalcemia. Suspect Wilson's disease if there are signs of liver failure, tremor, rigidity, and convulsions in a person under age 40. Also consider Cushing's syndrome, hypoglycemia, and hyper- and hypoparathyroidism.
- **Disorders of heart, lung, liver, and kidney:** Particularly CHF, arrhythmias, SBE, chronic hypoxia and hypercapnia (e.g., emphysema), hepatic encephalopathy, uremia, dialysis dementia.
- **Other:** Malnutrition (particularly vitamin B_{12} and folate deficiencies—check for pernicious anemia and combined system disease), remote effects of carcinoma, SLE, epilepsy.

DIFFERENTIAL DIAGNOSIS

Normal aging may mimic mild dementia, particularly if the patient is stressed by *environmental changes, social isolation, fatigue,* or *visual and hearing disorders* (sensory deprivation). Many elderly will develop mild *anxiety, depressive,* or *hypochondriacal* disorders that mimic dementia, but with persistent questioning and encouragement, normal memory, orientation, etc., can be seen. Intellectual deterioration with schizophrenia is differentiated from dementia by a history of psychosis and social withdrawal and by the presence of a characteristic thought disorder. An Amytal interview may help distinguish dementia from *catatonic schizophrenia.* In *delirium* there is an altered and fluctuating level of consciousness. **Delirium and dementia frequently coexist, but the delirium must clear before the diagnosis of dementia can be made.**

A *major depression* is the most common cause of *pseudodementia.* Unlike the demented patient, these patients have a rapid recent onset (family can usually date it), *complain* of a severe memory loss (usually mild when tested), have marked affective changes, emphasize their inabilities and failings, and frequently answer simple questions with "I don't know" (the demented patient usually attempts an answer). A temporary clearing during an interview and the lack of a deteriorating course helps identify these patients. Consider a DST and MRI. These patients usually improve with antidepressants or ECT.

Do not mistake an aphasia due to a focal lesion for a dementia (although perhaps 10% of severely demented patients have a related aphasia).

TREATMENT

Supportive Treatment

- Provide good physical care, e.g., good nutrition, eye glasses, hearing aids, protection (e.g., stairs, stoves, medication), and so on. Physical restraint is necessary at times.
- Keep in familiar settings, if possible. Surround with familiar objects; keep old friends engaged. Encourage the family's participation and understanding.
- Keep the patient involved—through personal contact, frequent orientation (remind them of the day, of the time). Dis-

cuss the news. Use calendars, radio, television. Structure daily activities—make them predictable.
- Help maintain patient's self-esteem. Treat him like an adult. Plan toward his strengths. Be accepting, tolerant.
- Avoid dark, isolated settings; avoid overstimulation.

Symptomatic Treatment

Psychiatric conditions may require *small* doses of appropriate medication (8,9).

- Acute anxiety, restlessness, aggression, agitation: for example, haloperidol 0.5 mg PO tid (or lower); risperidone 1 mg PO daily. Stop after 4–6 weeks.
- Nonpsychotic anxiety, agitation: e.g., diazepam 2 mg PO bid; venlafaxine XR. Stop after 4–6 weeks.
- Chronic agitation: SSRIs (e.g., fluoxetine 10–20 mg/day) and/or buspirone (15 mg bid); also consider low-dose β-blockers.
- Depression: consider SSRIs and other new antidepressants first; with TCAs, begin slowly and work up to—e.g., desipramine 75–150 mg PO daily).
- Insomnia: for short periods only; use (e.g.) temazepam 15 mg PO HS.

Specific Treatment

- Identify and correct any treatable condition.
- No specific drug treatment for dementia has been found to be consistently useful, although many are being investigated (e.g., cerebral vasodilators, anticoagulants, cerebral metabolic stimulants, stimulants, hyperbaric oxygen). Vitamin E (an antioxidant) is being investigated as a possible agent to slow the progression of AD. Increasing central cholinergic activity may provide temporary relief of some symptoms in a few patients with AD.

Tacrine (Cognex, THA, or tetrahydroaminoacridine), a reversible synthetic acetylcholinesterase inhibitor, increases acetylcholine and may produce modest cognitive improvement in moderate dementia (10). Begin at 40 mg and raise by 40 mg every 6 weeks until at 160 mg. Thirty percent have increased liver enzymes (ALT > 3 times nl); stop if ALT is > 5 times nl. Pancreatic inflammation, nausea, vomiting, and diarrhea can also be problems. A newer promising cholinesterase inhibitor is donepezil (Aricept; 5–10 mg QD), which does not seem to pose the risk of liver damage (but still produces GI distress).

REFERENCES

1. Corey-Bloom J, Thal LJ, Galasko D, et al. Diagnosis and evaluation of dementia. *Neurology* 1995;45:211–218.
2. van Leeuwen FW, de Kleijn DPV, van den Hurk HH, et al. Frameshift mutants of amyloid precursor protein and ubiquitin-B in Alzheimer's and Down patients. *Science* 1998;279:242–247.
3. Folstein MF, Folstein SE, McHugh PR. Mini-Mental State—a practical method for grading the mental state of patients for the clinician. *J Psychiatr Res* 1975;12:189–198.
4. Rouleau I, Salmon DP, Butters N. Longitudinal analysis of clock drawing in Alzheimer's disease patients. *Brain Cogn* 1996;31:17–34.
5. Terry RD, Katzman R, Bick KL. *Alzheimer disease.* New York: Raven Press, 1994.
6. Stern RG, Mohs RC, Davidson M, et al. A longitudinal study of Alzheimer's disease. *Am J Psychiatry* 1994;151:390–396.
7. Evans DA, Beckett LA, Field TS, et al. Apolipoprotein Eε4 and incidence of Alzheimer disease in a community population of older persons. *JAMA* 1997;277:822–824.
8. Flint AJ, Van Reekum R. The pharmacologic treatment of Alzheimer's disease: a guide for the general psychiatrist. *Can J Psychiatry* 1998;43:689–697.
9. Kunik ME, Yudofsky SC, Silver JM, et al. Pharmacologic approach to management of agitation associated with dementia. *J Clin Psychiatry* 1994;55[Suppl 2]:13–17.
10. Conway EL. A review of the randomized controlled trials of tacrine in the treatment of Alzheimer's disease. *Clin Neuropharmacol* 1998;21:8–17.

Chapter 7

Suicidal and Assaultive Behaviors

THE SUICIDAL PATIENT

Epidemiology

- Reported suicides in the United States are 31,000/yr (12/100,000; 300,000 attempts annually).
- Suicide is underreported and often listed as accidental.
- Attempted suicide: successful suicide ratio = 10–20:1.
- Suicide increases with age; the third leading cause of death in male adolescents and college students.
- Completers 3:1 (M:F); attempters 3:1 (F:M).
- Most common attempt is by drug ingestion; most likely to be fatal is by shooting.
- Most patients are *not* psychotic or incompetent; most *are* depressed.

All clinicians will encounter suicidal patients. Many will not recognize them. Some of those patients will kill themselves.

Identifying the Potentially Suicidal Patient

One fifth of suicides are unanticipated. Accurate prediction is difficult, if not impossible, with present knowledge. Entertain the possibility when (1)

1. The patient has made a suicide attempt (seen in the ER, medical ward, etc.);
2. Overt or indirect suicide talk or threats: "You won't be bothered by me much longer" (most often made to family members);

3. Depressed or anxious mood due to an observable depression;
4. Significant recent loss (e.g., spouse, job, self-esteem);
5. Unexpected change in behavior: making a will, intense talks with friends, giving away possessions;
6. Unexpected change in attitude: suddenly cheerful, angry, or withdrawn.

Assessing Suicidal Risk

Assessment Procedure

First, build rapport during a supportive nonjudgmental interview. If not volunteered, investigate suicidal thoughts by asking questions of increasing specificity, e.g., "Have you been feeling sad?" "Have you thought of doing away with yourself?" "How?," etc. Asking about suicide does not precipitate it. After a serious attempt, wait until the patient is alert enough to cooperate. Always ask about suicidality during a psychiatric assessment.

The following must be learned about *all* suicidal patients:

1. The patient's intention—why does he or she want to die?
2. Is a suicide plan made?—the more specific the plan, the more likely the act.
3. Method—the more lethal the technique, the more serious the plan.
4. Presence of psychiatric or organic factors—e.g., psychotic depression, thought disorder, sedative self-medication, organicity.
5. Determine the role of impulsivity versus premeditation.
6. Is the precipitating crisis resolving?
7. Take an "inventory of loss."
8. Does the patient have plans for the future?
9. Does the patient have caring family or other supports?
10. Does the patient think she is going to commit suicide?

Population Risk Factors
- Males
- Elderly
- Isolated individuals
- Whites
- American Indians
- Policemen

Individual Risk Factors

- Sense of **hopelessness** [*particularly* in a patient with major depression (2)], helplessness, loneliness, exhaustion, "unbearable" psychological pain.
- Psychiatric illness (3) (in 90% of suicide patients), mainly:
    (1) **Major mood disorder** (either 1° or 2°; 50% of all suicides), particularly with vegetative signs or constriction of thought; 15% lifetime suicide risk.
    (2) **Alcoholism** (suicide rate 50 times normal—25% of all suicides)—mostly chronic patients, mostly men, often after interpersonal loss, 3%–4% lifetime risk. Much higher if also depressed and with poor social supports (i.e., many patients). Drug addiction (10% die by suicide).
    (3) **Schizophrenia,** particularly when lonely, depressed, chronic, or with persecutory delusions or self-destructive command hallucinations; 10% or more lifetime risk.
    (4) Other: Psychoses due to organic conditions; personality disorders (borderline, antisocial), panic disorder with comorbid depression.
- Failing health, particularly if previously independent (5% of all suicides); chronic medical impairment; HIV/AIDS.
- Intoxication; active use (abuse) of *alcohol* and drugs.
- Impaired impulse control for any reason; hostility.
- **Past history of suicide attempts,** particularly serious attempts.
- Nature of past or present suicide attempts, e.g., shooting or jumping more lethal than most ingestions or wrist cutting. Warning given? Help available at the time?
- Family history of suicide; personal exposure to suicide; suicide itself may run in families genetically.
- Widowed, divorced, separated, *single, unemployed,* retired.
- Medical patients on renal dialysis.
- Family stresses or instability; few external supports.
- A change in status—*up* or down.
- Recent loss or rejection.
- Parental loss during childhood.

Other Risk Factors

- Holidays, spring, anniversaries.
- Possible biochemical measures of suicide potential (4): decreased CSF 5-HIAA and HVA and increased MHPG;

decreased urine NE/E ratio; increased adrenal weight; positive DST.

Initiating Appropriate Treatment

The first question often is "Should you hospitalize?" If the patient has pressing suicidal thoughts and/or decreased impulse control coupled with several risk factors, hospitalize, if only overnight. Be conservative. Do not write off patients as "just manipulative"—all statements of suicide intent initially should be taken seriously (particularly from adolescents). Manipulative suicide patients have "accidentally" killed themselves after being denied admission— 60% of successful suicides have had previous suicide attempts. The most emotionally upset patient is not necessarily the most suicidal. The suicidal state is episodic; a patient may be "safe" just hours after a serious suicide attempt. Be very cautious of the patient who has trouble considering any alternative to suicide.

The decision *to* hospitalize should be communicated to the patient decisively but optimistically. Hospitalization should be involuntary if necessary. Ensure the patient's physical safety in the hospital through appropriate "suicide precautions" (e.g., close supervision, no isolation, no dangerous objects).

A patient of lesser risk may be followed as an outpatient if there is a reliable family to help monitor them—assess that support. If the patient is *not* to be hospitalized, specific plans for follow-up must be made with the patient. Be absolutely clear about this with him or her.

Treatment Principles

1. Identify and treat psychiatric or medical conditions. Treat depression vigorously. Treat psychotic depressions with an antidepressant *and* antipsychotic. If the patient is determinedly suicidal, use ECT rather than wait for a medication response. Antipsychotics and benzodiazepines may be briefly useful with the agitated patient.
2. Develop a therapeutic alliance with the patient. Be concerned and accepting. Attempt to understand why the patient wants to die. Allow the patient to express anger, "unacceptable" thoughts, and feelings of rejection and hopelessness. These patients often feel misunderstood and trapped but unable to ask for help. Reduce the psychological pain any way you can.

3. Suicidal patients are usually *ambivalent about death* and may not know why they are trying to kill themselves. Point out that ambivalence to them—show them evidence of their desire to live. Be hopeful. Be definite. Make specific plans with and for the patient. Appeal to his or her mature rather than regressive side.
4. The patients are often bewildered and have a narrowed focus of thought—deal with reality issues.
5. Do not minimize the seriousness of a suicide attempt to the patient.
6. Never agree to hold a suicide plan in confidence.
7. Help the patient to grieve over losses.
8. Do not explain away the patient's symptoms (e.g., "I'd feel the same way myself").
9. Suicide potential can change rapidly. Reassess the patient's state of mind frequently.
10. Use community resources. Involve the family and significant others in treatment; use family therapy when appropriate. Actively try to reduce social isolation and withdrawal. Help make changes in the patient's environment where it is pathologic.
11. Many suicides in depressives occur during the first 3–6 months after hospital discharge. *Do not lose contact* with the patient. Monitor closely during holidays.
12. Be active but insist that the patient ultimately take responsibility for his or her own life.
13. Tricyclics, monoamide oxidase inhibitors, and many sedative-hypnotics have serious overdose potential. Some depressed outpatients store medication, so track drugs prescribed. If an antidepressant is required, use a newer safer one.

Theoretical explanations of suicide include the loss of a sense of identity with the social group (Durkheim), hostility turned against the self (Freud), a "cry for help," and a reflection of biologic psychiatric conditions.

THE VIOLENT PATIENT

Human aggression has complex and uncertain biologic, psychosocial, and cultural roots. Implicated in violent behavior are lesions of the prefrontal cortex (frontal lobe syndrome) and stimulation of the amygdala and limbic system (5). Also, find elevated androgens and CSF norepinephrine or decreased CSF serotonin (similar to "violent" suicide) and GABA (6,7).

Prediction of violence is difficult. Anyone can become violent, yet some *groups* are at risk: young males aged 15 to 25; urban, black, and/or violent cultural subgroups; and alcoholics. Key *individual* predictors of violent behavior are

1. A past history of violence;
2. Active use of alcohol;
3. Physical abuse as a child;
4. Some form of brain injury.

Mental Disorders with Associated Violent Behavior

Although most mentally ill are not dangerous, some patients present an increased risk. (Note: Serious medical illness can first present with violent behavior.)

1. Organic brain syndromes—particularly with confusion or decreased impulse control (e.g., the demented, drugs in the elderly, hypoglycemia, CNS infections, anoxia, metabolic acidosis).
2. Alcohol and drug abuse—particularly with intoxication, delirium, or delusional states of Etoh, amphetamines, cocaine, or PCP; also with intoxication from inhalants or "downers."
3. Schizophrenia, paranoid and catatonic types—particularly with command hallucinations or patients who drink.
4. Acute psychotic states of any origin.
5. Certain mentally retarded; XYY karyotype (possibly), and others.
6. Severe attention deficit disorder with hyperactivity, in adults.

Several Recognizable Patterns of Violence

1. **Chronic, aggressive, self-aggrandizing lifestyle:** Seen with **ANTISOCIAL PERSONALITY DISORDER** and thus associated with drug and alcohol abuse, onset in youth, delinquency and adult crime, truancy and school failure. Patients fight frequently and are "constantly in trouble." Serious affective disorders are common in this population.
2. **Episodic violence:** Explosive rages with little provocation, daily to several times a year, brief occasional amnesia for

event and remorse about it. A mixed group of clinical presentations; CNS abnormalities in most. If violence is *directed,* consider

- **INTERMITTENT EXPLOSIVE DISORDER** (DSM-IV p. 612, 312.34)—usually males with history of violent outbursts and numerous axis I problems, including mood disorders (8,9), family history of violence, neurologic soft signs, abnormal EEGs. Normal between episodes
- **PERSONALITY CHANGE DUE TO A GENERAL MEDICAL CONDITION, Disinhibited Type** (DSM-IV p. 173, 310.1)—neurologic origin (encephalitis, epilepsy, MS, tumor, poststroke, etc.), disturbed personality between episodes
- Rages in borderline or histrionic personality disorders, particularly when intoxicated.

If violence *poorly directed,* consider temporal lobe epilepsy (get NP leads), alcohol idiosyncratic intoxication, or other neurologic syndromes.

Evaluating Threats of Violence

Take all ideas or threats of violence seriously. Assess risk factors. What is the patient's current mental state? Can he or she control impulses and rage? Does the patient feel under great tension and fear losing control? Is there an intended victim? Is the victim covertly provoking the attack? Specific plans made? Sadistic fantasies present? Weapons available? Patient armed (always check)? Family support system present?

Management of the Acutely Violent Patient

1. First decide if the patient is acutely out of control. If so, treat immediately with restraint and medication, not talk. See immediately—do not keep him or her waiting.
2. Approach an unfamiliar patient cautiously and from a position of strength (help available, open door). Be alert to warning signs (e.g., restless, demanding). If talking appears useful, try, but set clear limits during interview. Use physical controls if patient cannot maintain control but emphasize their temporary helping nature. If patient arrives in restraints, *do not*

remove until rapport established and some evaluation done; however, many patients do better without restraints. Restraints may increase agitation and cause hyperthermia. If force is needed to subdue, use overwhelming force—one person to each limb. Do not take chances.

3. Medication for most acutely agitated patients: *lorazepam*, 1–2 mg IM (well absorbed IM) q 2–4 hours, maximum of 3 doses; *haloperidol* 5 mg IM hourly for 3–4 doses; or droperidol (5 mg IM hourly for 2–3 doses—not approved by the FDA for that purpose, however). Has patient taken CNS depressants, is he delirious, or is a medical condition responsible for behavior? If so, hold medications and observe. ECT can control psychotic violence.

4. If patient is threatening and agitated but not wild, treat with respect—be civil, direct, confident, calm, reassuring. Do not challenge, provoke, or openly disagree with the patient. Eliminate red tape. *Always* explain what you are doing, and why. Violent patients are often frightened—find out why and of what.

5. Determine etiology of violence. Is a mental illness present? A brain injury? Drugs involved (get urine screen)? Are there identifiable environmental precipitants? Expect to intervene directly with the psychotic patient.

6. Most patients can be "talked down" with support, understanding (and medication); however, hospitalize involuntarily if necessary. Is this really a criminal matter, and should the police be involved instead?

Ongoing Care

1. The chronically violent patient should receive medication trials. Treat psychosis with antipsychotics, and seizures with anticonvulsants. For continued aggression, consider (10,11)
   - Clozapine or risperidone (preferred for hostile schizophrenics);
   - SSRIs [e.g., fluoxetine (12)] for a variety of conditions and buspirone (head injury, mental retardation);
   - Propranolol (200–800 mg/day, divided doses), nadolol (up to 120 mg/day), or pindolol; may take 4–6 weeks for effect;

- Carbamazepine (600–1,200 mg/day, divided doses), valproic acid, and lithium (blood level 0.6–1.2 mEq/L) *may* be useful in violent patients with bipolar disorder, schizophrenia, mental retardation, intermittent explosive disorder, and other stimulants in hyperactive adults;

  Benzodiazepines can be useful during times of stress, but paradoxical rages occur in some patients.

2. Teach the patient to recognize early signs of increasing anger and to develop ways to discharge tension. The severely brain damaged may need a structured environment and behavioral techniques.

3. Help the patient develop a support system and learn to control environmental stresses. Maintain a channel of communication with the potentially violent patient—be available by phone. Also, you have some legal responsibility.

REFERENCES

1. Goldstein RB, Black DW, Nasrallah A, et al. The prediction of suicide. *Arch Gen Psychiatry* 1991;48:418–422.

2. Mendonca JD, Holden RR. Are all suicidal ideas closely linked to hopelessness? *Acta Psychiatr Scand* 1996;93:246–251.

3. Beautrais AL, Joyce PR, Mulder RT, et al. Prevalence and comorbidity of mental disorders in persons making serious suicide attempts. *Am J Psychiatry* 1996;153:1009–1014.

4. Arora RC, Meltzer HY. Serotonergic measures in the brains of suicide victims. *Am J Psychiatry* 1989;146:730–736.

5. Krakowski M. Neurologic and neuropsychologic correlates of violence. *Psychiatric Ann* 1997;674–678.

6. Niehoff D. *The biology of violence.* New York: The Free Press, 1999.

7. Volavka J. *Neurobiology of violence.* Washington, DC: American Psychiatric Press, 1995.

8. Coccaro EF, Kavoussi RJ, Berman ME, et al. Intermittent explosive disorder-revised: development, reliability, and validity of research criteria. *Comp Psychiatry* 1998;39:368–376.

9. McElroy SL, Soutullo CA, Beckman DA, et al. DSM-IV intermittent explosive disorder: a report of 27 cases. *J Clin Psychiatry* 1998;59:203–210.

10. Citrome L, Volavka J. Psychopharmacology of violence, part II. *Psychiatric Ann* 1997;27:696–703.

11. Ratey JJ, Gordon A. The psychopharmacology of aggression. *Psychopharmacol Bull* 1993;29:65–73.
12. Fuller RW. The influence of fluoxetine on aggressive behavior. *Neuropsychopharmacology* 1996;14:77–81.

Chapter 8

Anxiety Disorders

Anxiety is ubiquitous; anxiety disorders are not. *Anxiety* is an unpleasant and unjustified sense of apprehension often accompanied by physiologic symptoms, whereas *anxiety disorder* connotes significant distress and dysfunction due to the anxiety. An anxiety disorder may be characterized by only anxiety, or it may display another symptom such as a phobia or an obsession and present anxiety when the primary symptom is resisted. *Fear* is also universal and can produce the symptom picture of acute anxiety states, yet in contrast to anxiety, the cause is obvious and understandable. A feature common to all the anxiety disorders is the unpleasant and unnatural quality of the symptoms (anxiety, phobia, obsession)—they are *ego alien* or *ego dystonic*. These tend to be chronic relapsing conditions—be alert for suicide.

Anxiety is mediated through a complex system that involves (at least) the limbic system (amygdala, hippocampus), thalamus, and frontal cortex anatomically and norepinephrine (locus ceruleus), serotonin (dorsal raphe nucleus), and GABA (GABA$_A$ receptor coupled with the benzodiazepine receptor) neurochemically. We do not yet know how these parts work.

CHRONIC MILD ANXIETY

Tension, irritability, apprehension, and mild distractibility are common (particularly in medical and psychiatric patients), often related to environmental factors, and treated with supportive and reality-oriented therapy. Medications are of little value chronically, whereas iatrogenic addiction is a serious problem. Environmentally induced, short-lived, mild anxiety (**ADJUSTMENT DISORDER WITH ANXIETY,** DSM-IV p. 626, 309.24) usually resolves with the disappearance of the stress.

CHRONIC MODERATELY SEVERE ANXIETY

A diagnosis of **GENERALIZED ANXIETY DISORDER** (GAD) (DSM-IV p. 435, 300.02) is made with more severe chronic anxiety (longer than 6 months; usually years, but waxing and waning) and including symptoms such as autonomic responses (palpitations, diarrhea, cold clammy extremities, sweating, urinary frequency), insomnia, poor concentration, fatigue, sighing, trembling, hypervigilance, and/or marked apprehension. It tends to run in families, has a moderate genetic component, and is associated with simple and social phobias and with major depression (40% or more of patients at some time; elevated risk for suicide) (1). Usually no obvious etiologic stress is found, but look anyway.

Consider both medication and psychotherapy. A new antidepressant, venlafaxine XR, seems to be particularly effective and safe for treating GAD (2). Use benzodiazepines sparingly (diazepam, 5 mg PO tid-qid or 10 mg HS) and for short periods (weeks to several months); allow medication use to follow the fluctuating course of the illness. Consider *buspirone* for a first medication or for chronic use (20–30 mg/day in divided doses). A patient may not find it effective after the "instant relief" of a benzodiazepine. Tricyclic antidepressants, SSRIs, and MAOIs are useful in selected patients (particularly those who have depressive sxs), whereas some patients with autonomic symptoms improve with β-blockers (e.g., propranolol 80–160 mg/day).

Encourage self-reliance, maintenance of productive activity, and reality-based cognitions. Train the patient in relaxation techniques (e.g., biofeedback, meditation, self-hypnosis). Over 50% of patients become asymptomatic with time (months, years), but the rest retain a significant degree of impairment. Help the patient understand the chronic nature of the illness and the likelihood of having to live with some symptoms (3).

ACUTE ANXIETY: PANIC ATTACKS

A **PANIC DISORDER WITHOUT AGORAPHOBIA** (DSM-IV p. 402, 300.01) has dramatic acute symptoms lasting minutes to hours, is self-limited, and occurs in patients with or without chronic anxiety. Symptoms are perceived by the patient as medical and are characteristic of strong autonomic discharge—heart pounding, chest pains, trembling, choking, abdominal pain, sweating, dizziness—as well as disorganization, confusion, dread, and often a sense of impending doom or terror. Attacks may come "out of the blue" or may be initiated by crowds, stressful situations, or anticipation ("anticipatory anxiety"). They may be repeated several times daily, weekly, or monthly and often disappear for months at a time (but may become chronic). A typical panic attack can be produced in 50%–75% of patients with panic disorder (but not in normal subjects) by the intravenous infusion of sodium lactate or breathing CO_2. (Panic patients seem to be hypersensitive to a sense of breathlessness, whether chemically or environmentally produced.)

Like other anxiety conditions, it runs in families (15% or more of 1° relatives, 30% or more of monozygotic twins), is probably genetic, but no linkage to a particular gene has been found. It is comorbid with major depression (50%), suicide, social and specific phobias, and alcoholism (30%) (however, family members are at risk only for panic disorder and social phobia). It occurs in women more frequently than in men (2 : 1), particularly those who have had a disturbed childhood and early difficulty separating from their parents (separation anxiety disorder). In its milder forms, panic disorder tends to grade into GAD clinically, although it appears to be a distinct disorder. In addition, one-third of patients with panic also have agoraphobia (**PANIC DISORDER WITH AGORAPHOBIA,** DSM-IV p. 402, 300.21; see below): combined, these conditions afflict about 2.5% of the population. Patients often receive the million dollar workup for angina, thyrotoxicosis, or abdominal complaints. Effective treatment exists.

1. Medication is essential for panic disorder. Several effective drugs are available, although response to any one is unpredictable. Some patients respond to initial doses of medication with dysphoria or marked jitteriness, so start slowly. Consider
   A. SSRIs, but also other serotonergic drugs such as clomipramine (4).
   B. Tricyclic antidepressants (e.g., imipramine or desipramine, 150–300 mg/day); expect 2–3 weeks for response.

C. MAOIs (particularly phenelzine, 30–75 or more mg/day); effective with a broad spectrum of patients but may take 4–6 weeks for a response.

D. Clonazepam (1–5 mg/day, bid); sedative but looks promising.

E. Alprazolam (0.5–2 mg/day tid-qid); patients respond rapidly, but depression, potential addiction, and need for frequent doses can be problems.

F. Other medication occasionally effective include β-blockers (propranolol), carbamazepine (400–1,200 mg/day), valproate (500–3,000 mg/day), and verapamil (240–480 mg/day).

Typical practice is to maintain meds for 6 months after improvement, then slowly discontinue. Unfortunately, the relapse rate is high, and "half-dose maintenance" may work better.

2. Cognitive-behavioral therapy *should* be coupled with medication (see discussion under "Agoraphobia") (5). Supportive psychotherapy is of use acutely but does not correct the condition or prevent relapses.

ANXIETY WITH SPECIFIC FEARS: PHOBIC DISORDERS

Phobias are fears that are persistent and intense, are out of proportion to the stimulus, make little sense even to the sufferer, lead to avoidance of the feared object or situation, and when sufficiently distressful or disabling are termed a **PHOBIC DISORDER.** Common, mild, frequently transient fears (of the dark, heights, snakes) receive no diagnosis. Phobias may wax and wane over months or years and may disappear spontaneously, but serious cases may continue for decades and gradually take the form of a depressive disorder. The fears may generalize during their developing stages (e.g., fear of a store generalizes to the street in front of the store and then to the entire shopping area).

More than 12% of the population may have a phobic disorder in some circumstances, yet in less than 1% is it significantly disabling. Many begin suddenly in women from stable families and of ages 15–30. Anxiety with ruminations may dominate the day-to-day picture, or anxiety may occur only when the phobic object is encountered directly. Relief occurs with escape, thus reinforcing the avoidance pattern—a vicious cycle. Phobics are at risk to abuse alcohol and drugs as self-medication. Three subtypes have been identified, all of which have a moderate genetic component:

1. **AGORAPHOBIA WITHOUT HISTORY OF PANIC DIS-ORDER** (DSM-IV p. 404, 300.22): Multiple phobias with chronic anxiety—specifically fears of open and/or closed spaces, crowded places, unfamiliar places, being alone, and, more generally, of a loss of a sense of security. Many other fears and hypochondriacal concerns may be present, as well as multiple other symptoms including fainting, obsessional thoughts, depersonalization (feel unreal, detached), and derealization (feel surroundings are unreal). Depression is common. This is the most disabling phobic disorder.

   This may actually be a subset of panic disorder because *most* patients with agoraphobia also have panic attacks (**PANIC DISORDER WITH AGORAPHOBIA**). Typically, these combined patients develop their agoraphobia as an extension of a panic disorder, i.e., unpredictable *panic attacks* cause them to avoid public places for fear of having an attack (*anticipatory anxiety*) which then reinforces the behavior (*phobic avoidance*). This is even more disabling than agoraphobia alone. It most commonly develops during the 20s (F:M = 2:1). Genetics are similar to panic disorder (10% or more of 1° relatives are similarly affected).

2. **SOCIAL PHOBIA** (DSM-IV p. 416, 300.23): Fear of scrutiny from others during public speaking, using public lavatories, blushing, eating in public, etc. Typically begins during early adolescence and is found in 3%–4% of the population (F:M = 2:1). Some patients are troubled by *specific* and limited social activities, whereas others suffer from *generalized* social exposure. Marked general anxiety is common in severe cases: The patient controls by avoidance—can be socially crippling. Frequently associated with substance abuse and depression but do not mistake for the social withdrawal of primary depression, schizophrenia, or paranoid states. If symptoms have been present life-long, consider avoidant personality disorder.

3. **SPECIFIC PHOBIAS** (DSM-IV p. 410, 300.29): Monophobias—of animals, storms, heights, blood, needles, etc. Usually begin in childhood, are found in 10% or more of the population (more frequent among women), and have few associated symptoms or syndromes.

Treatment (2-Fold)

1. Cognitive-behavior therapy is essential in all three types of phobias (6). The key to treatment is **exposure** to the feared object or situation coupled with a reversing of the fearful expectations ("cognitions") about the upcoming encounter. *Systematic desensitization* (by reciprocal inhibition) uses a graded hierarchy of frightening stimuli, allowing the patient to "work up" to facing the phobic object. In *flooding,* the patient faces the feared object or situation directly, whereas with *implosion* the exposure is to the idea of the object or a vivid account of the "terrible" consequences expected. Social skills training may also be required for those who are socially inept. Such treatment may require (and be enhanced by) support and/or antianxiety medication.

2. Medication: Minor tranquilizers are used temporarily to help the patient confront the phobia. In social phobias, β-blockers (e.g., propranolol, atenolol) can be used to help control incapacitating autonomic symptoms (e.g., before a speech) if the symptoms are specific, whereas MAOIs (e.g., phenelzine), SSRIs, and gabapentin (Neurontin) are effective with generalized social phobias (7). In the agoraphobic, with or without panic attacks, use medication for panic disorder (TCAs, MAOIs, alprazolam). Once the panic attacks are controlled with medication, an agoraphobic usually needs supportive exposure to the feared situations (without experiencing panic) before the phobia resolves. "Half-dose" maintenance medication may be necessary as well.

POSTTRAUMATIC STRESS DISORDER (DSM-IV p. 427, 309.81)

If a patient suffers a severe loss or stress (e.g., rape, serious car accident, harm to a child or spouse, natural disaster, combat, prison camp, etc.), he or she may develop the clinical syndrome of **POSTTRAUMATIC STRESS DISORDER** (PTSD) (8). A mixture of the following symptoms are present initially (9)

- Marked anxiety;
- Personality change with irritability and poor concentration;
- An exaggerated startle response;
- Insomnia and nightmares;
- Intrusive thoughts of the event;

- Reliving the feelings experienced at the time;
- Avoidance of anything associated with the trauma;
- Emotional blunting, which can impair interpersonal relationships and day-to-day functioning.

Later, depression, emotional numbing, and preoccupation with the trauma may predominate. The more severe the stress, the more likely PTSD is (a) to develop and (b) to be long-lasting. It may resolve after months (lasts 1–3 months = *acute*) or, untreated, last for decades (>3 months = *chronic*). Occasional patients present primarily with physical symptoms or chronic pain. Comorbid psychiatric conditions include depression, anxiety and panic disorders, dissociative states, and substance abuse.

Patients with PTSD are more likely to have a personality disorder, a previous history of depression or substance abuse, a childhood history of physical abuse, or a family history of psychopathology, but presumably PTSD can occur in anyone who has experienced sufficient stress (found in 1%–9% of the general population; average = 3.6%; higher in special populations). Psychophysiologic arousal at the time of the stress seems to be important in developing PTSD, whereas conditioned arousal keeps it going.

PTSD patients are notoriously noncompliant: 70%–80% or more drop out of treatment, presumably because they cannot tolerate reliving the event in therapy. Medication is useful in many cases: benzodiazepines briefly for anxiety but primarily tricyclic antidepressants (imipramine 150–300 mg/day), MAOIs (phenelzine 45–75 mg/day), or SSRIs in moderately high doses. Carbamazepine has been found useful in controlling flashbacks, nightmares, and intrusive recollections (400–600 mg/day, 5–10 µg/mL), whereas propranolol (80–160 mg/day) may reduce sympathetic hyperarousal. Some clinicians argue that clonidine is the most effective medication for treating symptoms of hyperarousal and reexperiencing (10). Psychotherapy should accompany medication: primarily education, support, and cognitive-behavioral therapy. Many, but not all, experts believe that the patient should be engaged in treatment as soon after the incident as possible. (For example, the rape victim needs special and sensitive care—often in the ER—after the assault, for psychiatric as well as legal reasons. Many of her interpersonal relationships may have been altered by that episode. Work with the family—the married victim often needs to establish a new equilibrium with her husband.)

ACUTE STRESS DISORDER (DSM-IV p. 431, 308.3)

Acute stress disorder (ASD) is an expected reaction of anyone experiencing an adequately severe trauma, yet individuals require different amounts and types of stress to develop it. PTSD symptoms predominate: nightmares, reexperiencing the event, avoiding stimuli that remind one of the trauma, and symptoms of increased arousal such as irritability, hypervigilance, poor concentration, and marked startle response. In addition, patients may respond for several days with derealization, depersonalization, and as though they are in a daze.

Typically, ASD will disappear after 1 to 2 weeks (if that long), but if it lasts for longer than 1 month, the diagnosis needs to be changed to PTSD. The most useful therapy is to get the patient to come to terms with his or her acute stressor *as soon as possible* by having them "talk it through" and realize that life can return (and is returning) to normal. Sometimes it is necessary to use benzodiazepines briefly to facilitate this process. Failure to put the patient's trauma into perspective and get on with one's life all to often results in the development of PTSD.

ANXIETY DISORDER DUE TO A GENERAL MEDICAL CONDITION (DSM-IV p. 439, 293.89)

Medical conditions (most commonly cardiac disorders) can produce anxiety states, although often they generate no sense of apprehension or foreboding. If suggestive physical symptoms accompany anxiety, remember

1. Abnormal EKGs and heart sounds help identify cardiac symptoms (chest pain, palpitations) due to *angina* pectoris, prolapse of the mitral valve, and cardiac *arrhythmias* (e.g., PAT). *Mitral valve prolapse syndrome* (MVPS—midsystolic click, late systolic murmur, and echocardiographic findings) occurs with increased frequency (15%–40% or more) in patients with panic disorder; however, anxiety and panic disorders may *not* be increased in patients with MVPS. Thus, the relation between the two is not clear.

2. The apprehension and dyspnea associated with bronchial *asthma* or *COLD* ("pink puffers") usually has accompanying wheezing or characteristic spirometric and radiographic features.

3. Acute intermittent *porphyria*—anxiety with abdominal focus; look for fever, leukocytosis, pain in extremities, prior drug exposure, elevated urine porphobilinogen; Watson-Schwartz Test is positive.

4. Characteristic findings usually occur with *duodenal ulcer* (bleeding, relief of pain with food, persistent crater by x-ray, suggestive gastric analysis) and *ulcerative colitis* (bloody diarrhea, fever, weight loss, sigmoidoscopic findings) but without them, differentiation is sometimes difficult. *Internal hemorrhage* may be accompanied by pain and restlessness—the picture develops quickly.

5. The vertiginous anxious patient with *Meniere's disease* also has deafness, tinnitus, and nystagmus during the attack.

If there are no localizing features to the acute attack or if the anxiety is chronic, consider

6. *Hypoglycemia*—at times indistinguishable from chronic or acute psychogenic anxiety; obtain blood glucose at the time of the episode; 5-hour GTT.

7. *Hyperthyroidism*—anxiety symptoms occur with rapid onset type; skin warm and moist rather than cold and clammy; look for exophthalmos; get T_3, T_4; check for goiter; consider TRH stimulation test.

8. *Pheochromocytoma*—anxiety attacks with hypertension; visual blurring, headache, perspiration, palpitations; get 24-hour urinary VMA or free catecholamines.

Other medical conditions can produce an anxiety syndrome: intracranial tumors, menstrual irregularities, hypothyroidism, hyper- and hypoparathyroidism, postconcussion syndrome, psychomotor epilepsy, and Cushing's disease. Appropriate tests help differentiate.

SUBSTANCE-INDUCED ANXIETY DISORDER (DSM-IV p. 443)

Almost any drug of abuse can produce an anxiety syndrome on intoxication, whereas anxiety symptoms commonly predominate upon withdrawal from alcohol, hypnotic-sedatives, and cocaine.

Likewise, a number of medications can produce anxiety with use (e.g., antihypertensives and other cardiac drugs, thyroid, sympathomimetics and bronchodilators, anticholinergics, antiparkinsonian medications, lithium, and antipsychotics; see Chapter 13). Once the cause is identified and corrected, the anxiety usually promptly disappears.

ANXIETY WITH OBSESSIONS AND COMPULSIONS: OBSESSIVE-COMPULSIVE DISORDER (DSM-IV p. 422, 300.3)

Obsessions are repetitive ideas, images, and impulses that intrude upon a patient who feels powerless to stop them. They are unwanted, distressful, occasionally frightening or violent (e.g., the impulse to leap before a car; the thought that the patient may attack his or her spouse), and often impair functioning. The patient can ruminate endlessly ("Did I lock the door?"); most develop rituals or *compulsions* (counting, touching, cleaning) to ward off unwanted happenings or to satisfy an obsession (e.g., an obsession with dirt leading to handwashing rituals). Compulsions are thus obsessions made manifest and occur in 75% or more of obsessives. The performance of the ritual relieves the anxiety from the obsession temporarily. Thinking is often magical ("My son won't have an accident if I stamp each foot 30 times"), and the patient is aware of this (11–13).

Obsessive-compulsive disorder (OCD) afflicts 2.3% of the population (F:M = 1:1), presents varying degrees of severity, and is chronic, with some spontaneous cures. OCD patients suffer depressive feelings (80%), major depression (30%), and Tourette's syndrome (5%); 8% of first-degree relatives have OCD. First symptoms occur by the 20s in 75%, may begin suddenly or slowly, and often have an episodic course. The clinical picture may be dominated by the rituals, which require direct treatment.

The cause of OCD is unknown, but CNS serotonin neurons are implicated in some cases. Moreover, CNS damage (e.g., head trauma), the orbitofrontal cortex, caudate, neostriatum, globus pallidus, and thalamus play roles. There is an increase in anxiety disorders in family members (15%) but only slightly increased OCD.

Differential Diagnosis

Obsessive-compulsive problems are common in serious psychiatric illnesses. About 20% of serious depressions have obsessive symptoms (major symptoms and family history help to separate, and treatment may be identical). Schizophrenics have bizarre obsessions and are usually comfortable with them. (Be cautious: OCD can reach psychotic proportions, so do not overdiagnose schizophrenia.) Some organic conditions may present early with obsessions and compulsions.

Treatment

Medication substantially reduces symptoms in 60% or more and should be tried: *clomipramine* (Anafranil) is the first choice (150–250 mg/day), then fluoxetine (40–80 mg/day); later possibly augmented with buspirone (5–20 mg tid) or clonazepam (0.5–2.5 mg bid-tid). Behavior therapy should be considered an essential complement to medication. For ritualizers, use a combination of *exposure* to the feared situation and *response prevention* (blocking the compulsive behaviors). For patients with just obsessions, use *imaginal exposure* (mentally experiencing what "could happen") and *thought stopping* (the therapist, and then later the patient, interrupts obsessional thought with the shouted word "Stop!").

From the combination of medication and psychotherapy, expect moderate to significant improvement. Medication promotes rapid change, but exposure sustains that change and may make medication unnecessary long term. For the chronic, treatment-resistant, and disabled patients, consider very localized psycho-surgery: either cingulotomy or bilateral anterior capsulotomy.

REFERENCES

1. Judd LL, Kessler RC, Paulus MP, et al. Comorbidity as a fundamental feature of generalized anxiety disorders. *Acta Psychiatr Scand* 1998; 98[Suppl 393]:6–11.
2. Rudolph RL, Entsuah R, Chitra R. A meta-analysis of the effects of venlafaxine on anxiety associated with depression. *J Clin Psychopharmacol* 1998;18:136–144.
3. Lader MH. The nature and duration of treatment for GAD. *Acta Psychiatr Scand* 1998;98[Suppl 393]:109–117.
4. Bocola V, Trecco MD, Fabbrini G, et al. Antipanic effect of fluoxetine measured by CO_2 challenge test. *Biol Psychiatry* 1998;43:612–615.
5. Tsao JCI, Lewin MR, Craske MG. The effects of cognitive-behavior therapy for panic disorder on comorbid conditions. *J Anx Dis* 1998;12:357–371.

6. Shear MK, Beidel DC. Psychotherapy in the overall management strategy for social anxiety disorder. *J Clin Psychiatry* 1998;59[Suppl 17]:39–44.

7. Davidson JRT. Pharmacotherapy of social anxiety disorder. *J Clin Psychiatry* 1998;59[Suppl 17]:47–51.

8. Yehuda R. *Psychological trauma.* Washington, DC: American Psychiatric Press, 1998.

9. Tomb D. The phenomenology of post-traumatic stress disorder. *Psychiatr Clin North Am* 1994;17:237–250.

10. Friedman MJ. Current and future drug treatment for posttraumatic stress disorder patients. *Psychiatric Ann* 1998;28:461–468.

11. Hollander E, Stein DJ. *Obsessive-compulsive disorders.* New York: Marcel Dekker, 1997.

12. Jenike MA, Baer L, Minichiello WE. *Obsessive-compulsive disorders.* St. Louis: Mosby, 1998.

13. Swinson RP, Antony MM, Rachman S, et al. *Obsessive-compulsive disorder.* New York: Guilford, 1998.

Chapter 9

Dissociative Disorders

Dissociation is the splitting off of specific mental activities from the rest of normal consciousness, such as the splitting of thoughts or feelings from behavior (e.g., to daydream through a boring lecture and yet end up with a complete set of notes without being aware of having taken them) (1). Minor dissociation is a common human phenomenon (2). *Dissociative disorders* demonstrate severe dissociation that produces significant and diverse symptoms and impairs functioning. Such disorders are fairly common (10% lifetime risk), typically occur within the context of childhood physical and/or sexual abuse, and are frequently comorbid with major depression, somatization disorder, PTSD, substance abuse, borderline personality disorder, conduct disorder, and antisocial personality disorder (3).

AMNESIA

Organic processes (usually involving the temporal lobes) account for most cases of significant memory loss in adults. These processes include intoxication or withdrawal from drugs or alcohol, various dementias, acute or chronic metabolic conditions (e.g., hypoglycemia, hepatic encephalopathy), brain trauma (i.e., postconcussive amnesia), brain tumors (particularly in the temporal lobes), cerebrovascular accidents, epilepsy (particularly temporal lobe epilepsy), and various degenerative or infectious CNS diseases. Transient global amnesia (TGA) is a sudden, self-limited, massive loss of memory in middle-aged or elderly patients due to a temporary (presumably vascular) cause. Always look for an organic cause for amnesia first.

Loss of memory from psychological causes is **DISSOCIATIVE AMNESIA** (DSM-IV p. 481, 300.12). Usually there is sudden anterograde loss of emotion-laden information after a severe physical or psychosocial stress. It occurs most frequently in women in their teens or 20s or in men during the stress of war. The patient often appears confused and puzzled during the attack, but recovery is typically rapid, spontaneous, and complete. However, some people have amnesia, partial or complete, for past periods in their lives that may last for months or years. Hypnosis may help revive memories.

If, usually after an acute stress, the patient suffers a severe memory loss, leaves home, and acts like a different person, he has **DISSOCIATIVE FUGUE** (DSM-IV p. 484, 300.13). Although patients present themselves well to strangers, on questioning they are usually unaware of their previous (real) identity and may seem somewhat perplexed about their current personal identity. However, occasional patients function for long periods of time in complex roles, undetected. The return of old memories and the old identity usually occurs abruptly within hours or days but may not happen for months (or longer). Fugue is more common in alcohol abusers (4).

The differential diagnosis of both conditions includes

1. Various organic conditions (see above).
2. Psychiatric conditions—Amnesia may often accompany severe depressive or anxiety states. Somnambulism may superficially resemble some fugues but has marked clouding of consciousness. PTSD, somatoform disorders, and other dissociative states often include amnesia as well.
3. Malingering and secondary gain in patients with antisocial personality disorder.

Evaluate these patients with a careful history and physical examination, liver enzymes, blood alcohol level, and drug screen. Further evaluation may include a CT scan and a sleep-deprived EEG with NP leads. Are old skills preserved during the attack (uncommon in organic conditions)? Is there obvious secondary gain? Is there a personal or family history for mental illness or epilepsy? The Amytal interview is occasionally diagnostic—organic patients usually become more confused, whereas patients with psychological amnesia may have a return of memory.

DISSOCIATIVE IDENTITY DISORDER (DID) (DSM-IV p. 487, 300.14)

Formerly known as multiple personality disorder (MPD), patients with this dramatic disorder (e.g., *The Three Faces of Eve*) believe that they have at least two (and sometimes many) personalities within themselves (5–7). One of the personalities is usually dominant, yet any one of them may dominate from time to time. The patient's behavior is consistent with whatever personality is in "control" at that moment. Each personality may or may not be aware of the presence of the others.

This poorly understood (and hotly debated) psychiatric condition begins in childhood (likely in response to abuse), is more common among females (3–9:1), tends to be chronic, and is replete with multiple symptoms such as anxiety, depression with suicidal impulses and acts, trances and amnesia, a multitude of somatic complaints, substance abuse and other "misbehavior," and psychotic-like symptoms. Once considered rare, it may be relatively common, particularly in milder forms, and is frequently mistaken for the more flamboyant personality disorders (particularly borderline), somatization disorder, major depression, anxiety and panic disorders, and schizophrenia. In fact, DSM-IV criteria are often fulfilled for DID and several of these conditions as well.

Proper treatment *may or may not* center around a careful integration of the different personalities and personality fragments through 1–3 times per week psychotherapy and hypnotherapy over years. This may be the best treatment or it may worsen the condition by helping to generate inaccurate memories (8)—treatment remains uncertain (9,10). Once personalities have been integrated or fused (considered a "cure" by the therapist), stress can fragment the personality again (Eve of *The Three Faces of Eve* is a good example).

DEPERSONALIZATION DISORDER (DSM-IV p. 490, 300.6)

These patients experience periods during which they have a strong and unpleasant sense of their own unreality (depersonalization), often coupled with a sense that the environment is also unreal (derealization). The patient may feel mechanical and separated from his or her own thoughts, emotions, and self-identity. Although many people transiently experience this phenomenon in a mild form, the experience for those receiving a clinical diagnosis is much more intense and recurrent. An episode occurs suddenly (often during relaxation after stress); usually in persons in their teens or 20s; may last for minutes, hours, or days; and then gradually disappears. It may return many times over the years.

Psychotherapy has been of little value. Recently, however, anxiolytics and antidepressants (e.g., fluoxetine) have seen some success. Rule out the symptom of depersonalization that may accompany psychiatric disorders (e.g., schizophrenia, depression, anxiety disorders, and histrionic personality disorder) and organic conditions (e.g., delirium, temporal lobe epilepsy, drug and alcohol use, brain tumor).

REFERENCES

1. Coons PM. The dissociative disorders: rarely considered and underdiagnosed. *Psychiatr Clin North Am* 1998;21:637–648.
2. Ross CA, Joshi S, Currie R. Dissociative experiences in the general population. *Am J Psychiatry* 1990;147:1547–1552.
3. Allen JG, Smith WH. Diagnosing dissociative disorders. *Bull Menninger Clin* 1993;57:328–343.
4. Akhtar S, Brenner I. Differential diagnosis of fugue-like states. *J Clin Psychiatry* 1979;40:381–384.
5. Ross CA. *Dissociative identity disorder.* New York: Wiley, 1996.
6. Piper A. Multiple personality disorder. *Br J Psychiatry* 1994;164:600–612.
7. Putnam FW. *Diagnosis and treatment of multiple personality disorder.* New York: Guilford Press, 1989.
8. Kluft R. Current controversies surrounding dissociative identity disorder. In: Cohen LM, Berzoff JN, Elin MR, eds. *Dissociative identity disorder: theoretical and treatment controversies.* Northvale, NJ: Jason Aronson, 1995:370.
9. Chu JA. The rational treatment of multiple personality disorder. *Psychotherapy* 1994;31:94–100.
10. Spira JL, Yalom ID. *Treating dissociative identity disorder.* New York: Jossey-Bass, 1996.

Chapter 10

Grief and the Dying Patient

Everyone endures personal losses; many suffer chronic illnesses. Everyone dies. Physicians attend at all of these events and need to recognize normal and abnormal human responses to loss (grief reaction and unresolved grief), illness, and death.

GRIEF REACTION

Normal Grief

Symptoms

BEREAVEMENT (DSM-IV p. 684, V62.82) (grief, mourning) is a normal response to a significant loss (of spouse, parent, child—but also of health, limb, career, savings, status, etc.) (1). *Expect* to see it with major losses—be alert for future problems if the patient does not grieve (although 30% of widows mourn briefly and very little) (2,3). If a loss is obviously approaching, mourning may begin before the loss actually occurs (*anticipatory grief*). Symptoms associated with divorce may also be coded as **PARTNER RELATIONAL PROBLEM** (DSM-IV p. 681, V61.1).

Recognize grief by restlessness, distractibility, disorganization, preoccupation, "numbness," feelings of sadness, apathy, crying, anxious pining, a need to talk about the dead, and intense mental pain during the days, weeks, and months after a loss. Somatic distress is common and includes generalized weakness, a tightness in the throat, choking, shortness of breath, palpitations, headaches, and GI complaints. Do not be surprised if the patient displays marked but short-lived irritability, hostility, or anger toward you, others, or the dead (you did not "do enough," they do not "care enough," he died, etc.). This often alternates with listlessness, social withdrawal, depression, and feelings of guilt (about that which was left undone or could have been done differently). Patients become preoccupied with their loss. They constantly think about the dead and review past experiences, visit the grave, and may even briefly deny the death.

About 25%—35% of patients have symptoms that suggest a major depression: anorexia, feelings of worthlessness, impaired memory, suicidal thoughts, and hopelessness. Nearly 10% have delusional thoughts and/or hallucinations. Be careful not to "overread" temporary bizarre behavior in the bereaved. Some patients develop psychophysiologic disorders, hypochondriasis, major anxiety symptoms, or phobias. A few begin to drink too much, some deteriorate physically, and major psychiatric illnesses (e.g., acute schizophrenia) may be precipitated in those predisposed (e.g., positive family history). Moreover, bereavement has been associated with increased ACTH and cortisol, decreased immune function and natural killer cell activity, and an increased rate of heart disease and malignancy (4,5). Death from suicide and illness is increased during the first year after the loss.

Unresolved Grief

Loss not dealt with through a normal mourning process *may* produce chronic symptoms (6,7):

- **Prolonged grief:** Grief develops into a chronic depression or a subsyndromal depression that lasts for more than 1 year in as many as 30%. Lowered self-esteem and guilt tend to be prominent (8).
- **Delayed grief:** The patient who does not grieve at the time of a loss is at risk for later depression, social withdrawal, anxiety disorders, panic attacks, overt or covert self-destructive behavior, alcoholism, and psychophysiologic syndromes. Chronic anger and hostility, marked emotional inhibition, or distorted interpersonal relationships also may be displayed. Unresolved grief *may* be an unsuspected cause of psychiatric disability in many people—always inquire about a past history of significant losses.

- **Distorted grief:** Exaggerated (bizarre, hysterical, euphoric, or psychosis-like) reactions occur in a few patients that have the effect of postponing the normal grieving process. Alternately, the patient may present with physical complaints (e.g., pain or "chronic illness behavior") and may be mistaken for having a primary medical problem.

Persons at risk for developing an abnormal grief reaction include those who

1. Received little support or understanding from others after their loss (e.g., abortion, suicide, death of an illicit lover);
2. Are social isolates, either "psychological loners" or those without family or friends nearby—multiple strong supports help truncate the mourning process;
3. Are inhibited, compulsive, or uncomfortable with any form of emotion;
4. Have experienced *multiple* recent losses or a sudden, severe, unexpected loss;
5. Have unresolved past losses;
6. Had ambivalent feelings about the deceased when alive and have reacted to the death with guilt.

Treatment

Encouraging satisfactory mourning is an important activity for the physician.

- Encourage mourning. Say it is *okay*. Say it is *important* and necessary. Explain that the anguish undoubtedly experienced during this process is essential and curative. However, do *not* force the patient—let him or her set the pace.
- Help the patient identify and experience his emotions—sadness, hopelessness, despair, anxiety, fear, anger. Assure the patient that these are normal, expected, and understandable. Do not be embarrassed by these emotions yourself.
- Help the patient review the loss. Be an active listener. Ask for a description of the deceased—ask for particulars, details, shared intimacies, etc. Become a support.
- See the patient frequently. Be interested. Be available, particularly over time. Recognize and tolerate relapses. Be alert to the presence of anniversaries.

- Do *not* use medication to attenuate normal grief—help the patient work through the grief instead. Sleeping medication may be useful. If anxiety or restlessness is excessive, consider a temporary use of minor tranquilizers (e.g., diazepam 5 mg PO tid) *as therapy is begun.* Treat a major depression or psychosis with medication.
- Work with the family. Help develop a sympathetic support system. Mourners are social outcasts—help decrease "the social isolation of the bereaved." Self-help groups can be very valuable (e.g., groups of parents who have lost a child, etc.).
- Keep the mourner "involved in life"—slowly at first, but insist on increasing independence.

THE DYING PATIENT

Few patients stress physicians as much as those who are dying. This need not be. Even if little can be done to change a fatal outcome, *care*ful handling by the physician and crucial others can help turn a patient's death (whether expected or untimely) into a time of genuine relief, satisfaction, and (even) growth. When time is so limited, new realities and priorities emerge that must be dealt with if life is to be concluded satisfactorily (9).

Normal Responses in the Dying

The news that one is dying produces a special kind of grief reaction. A typical series of "stages" or psychological reactions to the threat of imminent death are seen frequently (10):

- **First Stage—Shock and Denial:** Denial is the initial reaction of many patients to being told that they are dying and is particularly severe in those "caught by surprise." They may refuse to believe the diagnosis, actively begin doctor shopping, or be dazed and appear oblivious to the significance of the diagnosis. This may be fleeting, but some patients may never pass beyond this stage.
- **Second Stage—Anger:** A frustrated, hopeless, angry, bitter, "Why me?" response often accompanies the realization of impending death. The anger is directed at the physicians (or family, God, fate, etc.) for the "unfairness" of this turn of events.

- **Third Stage—Bargaining:** The patient attempts to bargain with physicians or God for more time—promising good behavior, good intentions, etc., in exchange for "a chance to see my boy graduate from college" etc.
- **Fourth Stage—Depression:** The patient despairs and begins to grieve. Be alert to suicide, particularly in the irritable, demanding, agitated depression.
- **Fifth Stage—Acceptance:** The patient is quiet and resigned. He has little outside interests but seeks the presence of loved ones or a few close friends.

These stages are not necessarily stepwise and invariable. Just as often the person will shift back and forth between stages (e.g., from denial to anger and then back to denial), exhibit varying degrees of denial throughout, but gradually become more detached. The younger the adult, the more likely the stages are to be turbulent and the problems severe.

Specific psychiatric problems occur often and should be identified and treated:

1. Depression is common but not "normal"; thus, if a depression is not relieved by support and time, a major depression may develop. Consider treatment with antidepressants.
2. Organic brain syndromes (usually waxing and waning) develop frequently and can be frightening to patients. Help them see the disorders as separate from themselves—as just another thing to be experienced.
3. Acute anxiety is common but usually temporary, particularly if treated with medication.
4. Communication failures between the patient and loved ones are very common and troublesome—often taking the form of a "tyranny of silence" or a lack of understanding on either one's part about the distress of the other. These need to be dealt with directly.

Treatment

Telling the Patient
- Choose a quiet and private spot, be relaxed, sit down with the patient, and briefly reveal the diagnosis. Use the patient's response as an indicator of how much to tell.
- Patients need to know and need a chance to ask questions, but, most of all, they need someone (usually the physician,

but also spouse, pastor, etc.) *available*—someone to help them grieve.

- Be truthful (but allow them to deny if they insist on it) and realistically hopeful ("We will begin treatment. Sometimes remissions occur.", etc.). *Do not* encourage false hopes, but do not dwell on the fatal outcome.
- Strong negative reactions do occur. Sedation can be helpful temporarily.

Treating the Patient

- Be supportive, empathic, warm, a good listener, hopeful (e.g., about goals to be achieved before death), and available. Get to know the patient as a person—attention to exclusively medical matters is "dehumanizing." Be tolerant of ups and downs. Recognize that the patient may become hostile toward you—be patient.
- *Always* take your lead from the patient. Some days some topics are too stressful. Other days patients "have" to talk. Only force the issue if their denial, anxiety, or anger is seriously obstructing good care. Occasionally confrontation may be required.
- Make them comfortable. Treat pain aggressively—narcotics are okay. Attend fastidiously to basic physical needs. Make their room pleasant and cheerful.
- Certain fears are common and need to be looked for and dealt with, e.g., fear of pain, of physical dependency, of being isolated, of losing control (emotional and physical), of being helpless, of the unknown, of leaving loved ones to flounder (financially or emotionally).
- It is essential to help the patient "work through" the process of dying. Help him set new priorities and goals (e.g., get his affairs in order). Help resolve old problems and feel good about current relationships. Help him be responsible. Encourage the patient to consider not only how he will die but also how he will live out the rest of his life.
- Do *not* insist that patients march through the "stages of dying" in a set order and on schedule.
- Allow the patient "terminal dependency"—it is okay finally to regress.

Treating the Family

- Family members show many of the signs of grief. Like the patient, they also may be angry, hostile, or denying. They may need treatment—help *them* mourn.

- It is important to keep the family (i.e., loved ones) involved. Help the patient die "with their blessing."
- It can be enormously beneficial (to the patient, to the family) if the patient can be supportive to the family members in their grieving.

Treating the Staff
- Recognize that the physician, nurses, aides, etc., are all affected by death. Anxiety, intellectualization, avoidance, and grieving frequently occur among staff—do not let this stress impair care. Staff conferences to ventilate and explore these issues may help.

THE CHRONICALLY ILL PATIENT

Chronic illness is another form of stress that entails grieving. Like the dying patient, these patients may deny their illness, become angry and resentful, regress, or become depressed. Common to all these reactions is anxiety associated with a loss of health and attractiveness, a loss of self-esteem, and the threat of dependency or even death. Certain personality types are at risk (e.g., the narcissistic or the very independent). Treatment principles useful with the grieving or dying patient apply here as well.

REFERENCES

1. Parkes CM. *Bereavement: studies of grief in adult life.* New York: International Universities Press, 1972.
2. Marmar CR, Horowitz MJ, Weiss DS, et al. A controlled trial of brief psychotherapy and mutual-help group treatment of conjugal bereavement. *Am J Psychiatry* 1988;145:203–209.
3. Zisook S, Shuchter SR, Sledge PA, et al. The spectrum of depressive phenomena after spousal bereavement. *J Clin Psychiatry* 1994;55[Suppl 4]:29–36.
4. Spurrell MT, Creed FH. Lymphocyte response in depressed patients and subjects anticipating bereavement. *Br J Psychiatry* 1993;162:60–64.
5. Zisook S. *Biopsychosocial aspects of bereavement.* Washington, DC: American Psychiatric Press, 1987.
6. Rynearson EK. Pathologic grief: the queen's croquet ground. *Psychiatric Ann* 1990;20:295–303.
7. Prigerson HG, Bierhals AJ, Kasl SV, et al. Complicated grief as a disorder distinct from bereavement-related depression and anxiety. *Am J Psychiatry* 1996;153:1484–1486.

8. Barry MJ. Therapeutic experience with patients referred for pro-longed grief reaction—some second thoughts. *Mayo Clin Proc* 1981; 56:744–747.

9. Brown JH, Henteleff P, Barakat S, et al. Is it normal for terminally ill patients to desire death? *Am J Psychiatry* 1986;143:208–211.

10. Kubler-Ross E. *On death and dying.* London: Tavistock, 1970.

Chapter 11

Conditions that Mimic Physical Disease

It is essential to differentiate organic illness from psychogenic illness in patients complaining of physical symptoms. Patients with physical concerns in whom no medical illness can be found and/or who do not improve with treatment are common. These frustrating patients often exhaust one doctor after another and usually end up being labeled "hysterics" or "crocks." This occasionally angry response by the physician does a disservice to these patients because, although some may be consciously "faking it" (malingering), most patients have as yet undiagnosed organic conditions or have symptoms that are unconsciously and involuntarily produced.

There are several discrete involuntary psychiatric syndromes (somatoform disorders; see below) that mimic organic disease. These disorders have typical clinical presentations, family histories, recommended treatments, and likely prognoses.

Failure to identify an organic etiology for a physical symptom does not necessitate a diagnosis of a somatoform disorder or malingering; these are not diagnoses by exclusion but rather should be based on specific characteristics. Consider the following diagnoses in any patient with a poorly specified or uncertain medical condition.

1. Undetected Physical Illness

The possibility of an underlying unrecognized illness must continue to be considered throughout the course of diagnosis and treatment, however long. Follow-up studies find 15%–30% of conversion reaction diagnoses to represent misdiagnosed organic disease. Physical illness may produce symptoms that mimic a somatoform disorder or may predispose susceptible patients to develop concurrent psychiatric conditions (it's not "*either, or*"). Some patients with subtle CNS disease are at risk for conversion symptoms, so always carefully evaluate neurologically. The physical conditions commonly found (on follow-up) among these "false-positive hysterics" include

- CNS disease: particularly epilepsy, MS, and postconcussion syndrome but also CNS infections (e.g., encephalitis), dementia, brain tumor, and cerebrovascular disease.
- Degenerative disorders: of musculoskeletal and connective tissues, including SLE, polyarteritis nodosa, early rheumatoid arthritis, and myasthenia gravis.
- Others: syphilis, TB, hyper- and hypothyroidism, hyperparathyroidism, porphyria, hypoglycemia, duodenal and gallbladder disease, pancreatic disease, etc.

Be suspicious of any somatoform disorder that *develops late in life*—very unlikely. Psychological testing is of little help in differentiation; do not be misled by a "neurotic" picture on the MMPI into prematurely abandoning the search for a physical cause.

SOMATOFORM DISORDERS

2. Conversion Disorder (DSM-IV p. 457, 300.11)

A patient whose predominant problem is an obvious loss of function of some part of the nervous system that no identified organic pathology completely explains (conversion symptom) may have a conversion disorder. Conversion symptoms include

- Motor: paralysis, astasia-abasia, seizures, urinary retention, aphonia, globus hystericus ("lump in the throat" that prevents swallowing);
- Sensory: paresthesia, anesthesia, anosmia, blindness, tunnel vision, deafness;
- Other: unconsciousness, vomiting.

In addition, the particular symptom appears to serve one of two specific psychological purposes.

1. As *primary gain,* the symptom "buries" an unconscious mental conflict. An unacceptable painful thought is repressed, and the emotional energy is converted to a physical symptom. Usually the specific symptom "chosen" represents the conflict symbolically (e.g., the negligent mother of a burned child develops anesthesia over the corresponding part of her body).

2. As *secondary gain,* the symptom gets the patient something he or she wants (e.g., paralysis permits dependency on wife or justifies workman's compensation) or allows him or her to avoid something they do not want (e.g., seizures prevent a court appearance).

As obvious as these relationships may be to the observer, the patient is unaware of them (unconscious), and the patient does not grasp their significance, even if they are explained (lacks insight).

Diagnosis

In the apparent absence of organic pathology, it is necessary to identify features in addition to a presumed conversion symptom before making the diagnosis (1). Realize also that as many as 25% of patients with conversion disorders have associated organic pathology (e.g., epilepsy in a patient with pseudoseizures is common), so also investigate symptoms only partially explained by the physical abnormalities. Features associated with conversion disorders include

- The symptom occurs abruptly and frequently follows an acute stress.
- There is often a past history of the same or a different conversion symptom.
- The disorder usually is seen first during adolescence or in the 20s and in a person predisposed by a dependent, histrionic, antisocial, or passive-aggressive personality disorder.
- The patients often have associated moderate anxiety and depression.
- The patients are frequently immature, shallow, and demanding, although they tend to cooperate with examinations. They tend to have lower intelligence, limited insight, and lower socioeconomic status.
- Indifference to the symptom may be found (*la belle indifference*).

The individual neurologic symptoms may have some characteristics that distinguish them from those of an organic etiology. In general, they tend to be variable, atypical, and inconsistent with anatomy.

Conversion Seizures Seizures (2,3) are often atypical and bizarre (patient may laugh or cry throughout seizure). Only infrequently is there incontinence, cyanosis, physical self-harm, tongue biting, or complete loss of consciousness during the seizure. Good muscle tone is preserved during the typically brief postictal stage (arm dropped onto face may land lightly or miss the face altogether). The onset is usually dramatic, and seizures rarely occur when the patient is alone. Sit patient quickly upright—seizures often stop.

Conversion Unconsciousness The loss of consciousness is usually light and incomplete with the patient showing some awareness of environmental events, particularly when he or she feels unobserved. VS and reflexes are normal, and the patient usually responds to painful stimuli. The eyes are held tightly shut, and some movements may be purposive (e.g., move to keep from falling from examination table).

Conversion Paralysis The paralysis is often variable, even during one examination. Paralysis of one limb, part of a limb, or hemiparesis are most common, but the specific involvement is often inconsistent with anatomy, and the related changes (e.g., tone, etc.) are atypical. DTR changes are variable, and pathologic reflexes (e.g., Babinski) are not present. The paralyzed limbs often show little resistance to passive movement but resist the pull of gravity. If there is resistance to a forced movement, it tends to give way abruptly (vs. gradually as in organic conditions). There may be movement when startled by a painful stimulus. Palpate the antagonists—they often contract to simulate agonist weakness. There are usually associated conversion sensory changes.

Astasia-Abasia This exaggerated and bizarre conversion ataxia varies from moment to moment. The patient falls toward walls and people, rarely falls to the floor, and rarely hurts himself despite a dramatic presentation.

Conversion Sensory Changes These are often dramatic, sometimes vague, and usually inconsistent with anatomy (e.g., "stocking and glove" anesthesia, loss of *all* senses on one side or below a certain level on a limb, loss of which stops *exactly* at midline). Careful testing differentiates most cases.

Conversion Blindness Visual disturbances are usually blurring, double vision, or tunnel loss but may be total blindness. Response to a bright light (check with EEG) and avoidance of threatening objects are often inconsistent with the degree of presumed visual loss.

When the diagnosis is in doubt, a single dose of IV sodium amobarbital (Amytal) often temporarily removes the conversion symptom, thus clarifying the diagnosis. Slowly give a 10% solution IV (1 ml/min, maximum of 500 mg). When the patient's words begin to slur, stop administration and observe for disappearance of symptom.

Differential Diagnosis
- Carefully rule out physical illness.
- Some patients with conversion symptoms require a primary diagnosis of major depression or schizophrenia.
- Two somatoform disorders (see below) have features in common with conversion disorders: somatization disorder and psychogenic pain disorder.
- Differentiation from malingering is difficult (see below).

Treatment
Some patients have a short course and are "spontaneous cures"; a few may be chronic (e.g., some paralyzed patients actually develop contractures), but most improve over weeks or months. A physical process is later identified in a significant minority (25%).

It is uncertain what treatment is best (4). Long-term psychoanalysis appears to effect real change in a few but is not for most patients. Use minor tranquilizers if anxiety predominates. Behavior modification has had mixed success.

Crucial to any therapy is the formation of a supportive therapeutic alliance, but these patients are generally resistant to treatment. Direct confrontation about the "hysterical" nature of the symptom rarely works—the patient usually withdraws. Help the patient ventilate. Help the patient explore areas of stress in her life but relate that to symptoms only after an alliance has been formed. Gradually identify the symbolic nature of the symptoms, if present.

Work with the family. Help restructure the patient's environment to remove the secondary gain, if possible. Educate other involved medical personnel about the disorder—help them avoid countertherapeutic hostility.

3. Somatization Disorder (DSM-IV p. 449, 300.81)

This syndrome, historically called hysteria or Briquet's syndrome, has been refined in the last few years and may or may not be coequal to the traditional diagnosis of hysteria. The patients have *numerous* vague and dramatic physical symptoms (usually presented in a dramatic way) that typically involve several organ systems:

- Conversion symptoms of all types, including *neurologic;*
- Vague and ill-defined *pains;*
- Menstrual/*sexual* problems, inhibited orgasm;
- GI, GU, and cardiopulmonary difficulties;
- Poorly characterized altered states of consciousness.

The symptoms wax and wane but usually are presented forcefully by the patient, who insists on examination and treatment. These patients often receive multiple operations and are at risk for iatrogenically induced drug addiction.

Analytically oriented researchers argue that symptoms are produced when forbidden impulses are repressed and the emotional energy associated with those drives is converted (conversion) into a physical symptom. Although definitive information remains incomplete, features currently associated with Briquet's syndrome include

- A chronic condition beginning in adolescence or during the 20s;
- Occurs primarily in women (1% of all women);
- Anxiety, irritability, and depression are common; frequent suicide attempts (but few successful);
- Lower intelligence and lower socioeconomic groups;
- Frequent interpersonal and marital problems;
- Often previous or concurrent history of antisocial behavior and a poor school history;
- Patients may have histrionic, dependent, or antisocial personality disorder (5);
- First-degree female relatives have a 20% incidence of somatization disorder. First-degree male relatives have increased prevalence of alcoholism and antisocial personality disorder.

Somatization disorder is difficult to distinguish from malingering, and occasionally there are elements of both present (6). It is essential to rule out inconstant and confusing medical syndromes (e.g., SLE, acute intermittent porphyria, TLE, MS, hyperparathyroidism), although most can be differentiated from the full Briquet's syndrome (reliable diagnostic screening tests are available). Follow-up studies find few cases of undiagnosed organic illness (unlike conversion disorder). Rule out somatization in schizophrenia and depression.

Treatment

Treatment success is limited (7). Focus usually should be placed on management rather than cure. Develop a therapeutic alliance by being sympathetic and interested in the patient and her health but do not make that your exclusive focus. Gradually encourage an examination of the patient's general life problems and coping styles. Help the patient develop mature social, occupational, and intimate interpersonal skills. Treat depression and anxiety with medication, if indicated, but recognize the risk for addiction.

4. Pain Disorder (DSM-IV p. 461, 307.8y)

These patients (often women) experience pain for which no cause can be found. It appears suddenly, usually after a stress, and may disappear in days or last years. It is frequently accompanied by organic illness that, however, does not adequately explain the severity of the pain. This condition is very similar to conversion disorder, and the patients may differ only by experiencing pain rather than neurologic deficit as the predominant symptom. Treatments are also similar.

5. Hypochondriasis (DSM-IV p. 465, 300.7)

Although many people may mentally expand a minor symptom into a major physical illness (particularly during times of stress), they rarely become preoccupied with it and can easily be dissuaded when examination and laboratory tests are normal. The hypochondriac, on the other hand, may (a) be convinced he or she is ill, reject evidence to the contrary, insist on further tests and treatments, doctor shop, appear pleased only if assured of sickness, and eagerly seek additional medical attention or (b) be consoled temporarily when reassured but resurrect old or new symptoms in days or weeks (a variant of OCD?). This common chronic condition begins in adolescence or middle age, is common among the elderly, and is resistant to therapy (8,9). The patient rarely sees a psychiatrist but rather drifts from internist to surgeon to neurologist, etc.

The patient is hyperalert to symptoms and presents them in great detail during the history. These patients usually have some specific idea of "what the trouble is" and merely may want the physician to concur. Physicians frequently become angry and rejecting toward the patient, which leads to further "shopping around." In severe cases, the patient becomes an invalid.

Many of these patients display anxiety or depression. Hypochondriacal features occur frequently in serious psychiatric conditions like schizophrenia, major depression, dysthymic disorder, and organic brain syndromes. Rule out other somatoform disorders, chronic factitious disorder, and malingering (10).

Treatment is unpromising (11). Symptoms may disappear if an associated depression or psychosis is successfully treated. Do not expect a "cure" but rather work with the patient to help *control* the symptoms. Assure the patient that the problem is persistent but not debilitating or fatal. See the patient frequently for short periods of time. Assure the patient that you will be available if needed but schedule regular appointments (to be kept whether or not he or she is feeling ill). Consider giving a mild medication (e.g., antihistamine, vitamin) that can be a focus of attention during appointments and will be evidence that he or she is taken seriously. This form of palliation can restore the patient to functional health more readily than any definitive medical treatment.

6. Body Dysmorphic Disorder (DSM-IV p. 468, 300.7)

This disorder of young adults can be minor or incapacitating: Patients can become preoccupied with an imagined physical defect, which they feel negatively affects their appearance, and seek surgical correction or become socially withdrawn or even housebound. Although in its minor forms it is surprisingly common, little is known of its etiology, family patterns, biology, or treatment (12,13). It has some characteristics of OCD (14).

It occasionally reaches psychotic proportions. SSRIs may help some.

7. Undifferentiated Somatoform Disorder (DSM-IV p. 451, 300.81)

This residual category contains patients complaining of non-specific weakness, fatigue, and vague but incapacitating medical symptoms (GI, GU, etc.). They share elements of the other somatoform disorders but without adequate focus. Thoroughly evaluated and completely unexplained "chronic fatigue syndrome" patients belong in this category. These patients are not uncommon; treat similarly to hypochondriasis.

SIMULATION OF PHYSICAL SYMPTOMS

Two categories of patients *voluntarily* mimic physical symptoms (15).

8. Malingering (DSM-IV p. 683, V65.2)

These people knowingly fake symptoms for some obvious gain (16). They may be trying to get drugs, avoid the law, get a bed for the night, etc. Despite their physical complaints (17), they tend to be evasive and uncooperative during evaluation and therapy, and they avoid medical procedures. When exposed, they may angrily give up their symptoms and sign out AMA. Antisocial personality disorder and drug abuse are common associated conditions.

9. Factitious Disorder with Predominantly Physical Signs and Symptoms (DSM-IV p. 474, 300.19)

These patients also knowingly fake symptoms but do so for psychological reasons: They usually prefer the sick role and may move from hospital to hospital to receive care. They are usually loners with an early childhood background of trauma and deprivation. They are unable to establish close interpersonal relationships and generally have severe personality disorders. Unlike many malingerers, they follow through with medical procedures and are at risk for drug addiction and for the complications of multiple operations (18).

Both groups of patients can be difficult to distinguish from the somatoform disorders and from organic illness, yet careful and *repeated* examinations will usually uncover their deceptions. The most common presentations include

- Abdominal pain: May have an abdomen "like a railroad yard."
- Heart: Complains of pain. May induce arrhythmias with digitalis or produce tachycardia with amphetamines or thyroid.
- Bleeding: Patient may take anticoagulants or add blood from a scratch to laboratory samples.
- Neurologic: Weakness, seizures, unconsciousness—difficult to differentiate from conversion symptoms.
- Fever: Produced by manipulating the thermometer (e.g., hot coffee in the mouth).
- Skin: Look for lesions in a linear pattern in areas the patient can reach.

Although both groups produce symptoms consciously, they should be dealt with differently. The malingerer should be handled formally (and often legally). The patient with a factitious disorder should be treated sympathetically and every effort made to convince him or her to enter psychotherapy (difficult). Unlike the malingerer, these patients are unable to control their self-destructive behavior, and that should be tactfully pointed out to them.

REFERENCES

1. Sharma P, Chaturvedi SK. Conversion disorder revisited. *Acta Psychiatr Scand* 1995;92:301–304.
2. Bowman ES, Markand ON. Psychodynamics and psychiatric diagnoses of pseudoseizure subjects. *Am J Psychiatry* 1996;153:57–63.
3. Lesser RP. Psychogenic seizures. *Neurology* 1996;46:1499–1507.
4. Moene FC, Hoogduin KAL, van Dyck R. The inpatient treatment of patients suffering from (motor) conversion symptoms. *Intern J Clin Exp Hypnosis* 1998;46:171–190.
5. Stern J, Murphy M, Bass C. Personality disorders in patients with somatization disorder. *Br J Psychiatry* 1993;163:785–789.
6. Creed F, Guthrie E. Techniques for interviewing the somatising patient. *Br J Psychiatry* 1993;162:467–471.
7. Bass C, Benjamin S. The management of chronic somatisation. *Br J Psychiatry* 1993;162:472–480.
8. Barsky AJ, Fama JM, Bailey ED, et al. A prospective 4- to 5-year study of DSM-III-R hypochondriasis. *Arch Gen Psychiatry* 1998;55:737–744.

9. Escobar JI, Gara M, Waitzkin H, et al. DSM-IV hypochondriasis in primary care. *Gen Hosp Psychiatry* 1998;20:155–159.

10. Black DW. Iatrogenic (physician-induced) hypochondriasis. *Psychosomatics* 1996;37:390–393.

11. Barsky AJ. Hypochondriasis: medical management and psychiatric treatment. *Psychosomatics* 1996;37:48–56.

12. Phillips KA, McElroy SL, Keck PE, et al. Body dysmorphic disorder: 30 cases of imagined ugliness. *Am J Psychiatry* 1993;150:302–308.

13. Zimmerman M, Mattia JI. Body dysmorphic disorder in psychiatric outpatients: recognition, prevalence, comorbidity, demographic, and clinical correlates. *Comp Psychiatry* 1998;39:265–270.

14. Phillips KA. Body dysmorphic disorder: clinical aspects and treatment strategies. *Bull Menninger Clin* 1998;62:A33–A48.

15. Feldman MD, Eisendrath SJ. *The spectrum of factitious disorders.* Washington, DC: American Psychiatric Press, 1996.

16. Powell R, Boast N. The million dollar man. *Br J Psychiatry* 1993;162:253–256.

17. Bauer M, Boegner F. Neurological syndromes in factitious disorder. *J Nerv Ment Dis* 1996;184:281–288.

18. Boldstein AB. Identification and classification of factitious disorders: an analysis of cases reported during a ten year period. *Int J Psychiatry Med* 1998;28:221–241.

Chapter 12

Psychosomatic Disorders

There are two overlapping classifications here. A **PSYCHO-SOMATIC DISORDER** (not in DSM-IV) is a physical disease *partially* caused or exacerbated by psychological factors, whereas the new DSM-IV category, **PSYCHOLOGICAL FACTORS AFFECTING MEDICAL CONDITION** (DSM-IV p. 678, 316), broadly identifies those psychological and social factors that influence the development and maintenance of medical disease. Both classifications apply only to those conditions in which psychological and/or behavioral influence is of *major* significance (but be aware that *any* physical disease may be modified by psychological stress). Neither the term "psychosomatic" nor the DSM-IV category refers to (a) a physical symptom or clinical presentation caused by psychological factors for which there is no organic basis (e.g., conversion disorder, pain disorder, somatization disorder) or (b) a patient with knowingly spurious physical complaints (e.g., factitious disorder, malingering), but the DSM-IV condition does allow for physical complaints due to habit disorders (e.g., dyspnea due to excessive smoking, problems from obesity).

MECHANISMS OF DISEASE PRODUCTION

There are many specific diseases influenced greatly by the "psyche" (see below), but although much studied, the mechanisms by which the brain produces such organic pathology are unclear.

Psychological Mechanisms

Stress, either internal or external, is required but is much more likely to cause disease if

1. The stress is severe (e.g., death of a loved one, divorce or separation, major illness or injury, financial crisis, incarceration). Holmes and Rahe developed a ranked scale of stressful life events (rated by life change units—LCU) and found a close correlation between an event's stress (in LCUs) and the patient's likelihood of developing a physical illness.
2. The stress is chronic.
3. The patient perceives the stress as stressful.
4. The patient has an increased level of general instability (e.g., difficult job, troubled marriage, urban dweller, socially disrupted environment, etc.).

It was once thought (F. Dunbar) that *specific* superficial personality traits produced specific organic diseases (e.g., that there is a "coronary personality," an "ulcer personality," etc.). It was also held (F. Alexander) that *specific* deep and unconscious unresolved neurotic conflicts caused specific physical disorders. Currently, the specificity that is generally accepted associates the "type A" personality (i.e., sense of time urgency, impatience, aggressiveness, upward striving, competitiveness, tendency to anger when frustrated, and particularly a "cynical hostility") with coronary artery disease. More generally accepted are nonspecific hypotheses that link a wide variety of stresses to the development of disease in an individual placed at risk by one or more of the following:

1. A genetic susceptibility.
2. A degree of chronic debilitation, a current illness, or "an organ vulnerability."
3. A tendency to react to stress with anger, resentment, frustration, anxiety, or depression.
4. A "psychological susceptibility" (e.g., patient is pessimistic and "expects the worst" vs. being optimistic and actively working to overcome stress) (3).
5. An "alexithymic" personality (4) (e.g., a person who is in poor contact with emotions and has an impoverished fantasy life).

Physiologic Mechanisms

These mechanisms are poorly understood, and only the broad outline can be sketched. Stress is perceived cognitively (by the cerebral cortex) but once recognized is mediated primarily by the limbic system that, under chronic stress, constantly stimulates the hypothalamus and the vegetative centers in the brainstem. This stimulation produces a direct effect on the various organs by

1. Activation of the autonomic nervous system (sympathetic and adrenal medulla; parasympathetic).
2. Involvement of the neuroendocrine system, i.e., *releasing hormones* from the hypothalamus travel through the pituitary portal system to the anterior pituitary where they cause the release of the trophic hormones (e.g., ACTH, TSH, GH, FSH) that either act directly or release other hormones from the endocrine glands (e.g., cortisol, thyroxin, epinephrine, NE, sex hormones). These produce a variety of changes in structures throughout the body. In 1976, Hans Selye emphasized the central role of cortisol as a primary mediator of the body's stress response (general adaptation syndrome—GAS): If cortisol is released too chronically, various organs are damaged, producing psychosomatic diseases.

The details have yet to be worked out; there remain more questions than answers. The recently identified hormones, endorphins, may play a major role in stress response regulation. Central to all these physiologic systems is the concept of homeostasis—psychosomatic diseases occur when the body's "natural balance" is upset, particularly if it is chronically upset.

Although psychosomatic medicine has been concerned primarily with those diseases believed to be "psychosomatic," recently the concept has been broadened to include (or overlap with) the field of behavioral medicine. The essence of behavioral medicine is the application of behavior modification techniques derived from learning theory to various medical problems (e.g., chronic pain, hypertension and other psychosomatic diseases, habit disorders, etc.). Techniques used include behavioral self-management methods, biofeedback, hypnosis, and various relaxation procedures.

SPECIFIC PSYCHOSOMATIC DISORDERS

Although stress can increase the susceptibility to any disease and most diseases are currently viewed as multifactorially determined, those that most clearly have a major psychosomatic contribution include the following disorders.

Cardiovascular

Coronary Artery Disease
More common in "Type A" personalities. These patients have increased serum cholesterol, low-density lipoproteins, and triglycerides; also increased urinary 17-ketosteroids, 17-hydroxycorticosteroids, and NE. Sudden death by MI is increased in patients experiencing a severe recent loss (first 6 months). Likewise, depression is correlated with increased risk for heart disease (5).

Hypertension
Chronic psychosocial stress *probably* plays a role in its development in genetically predisposed patients. The mechanism is uncertain but may not be related to the brief hypertension that occurs during periods of acute stress. May occur more frequently in Type A people and in compulsive people who "store resentment" and who handle angry feelings poorly. Treat first with antihypertensives. Relaxation therapy (e.g., progressive relaxation, meditation, hypnosis) is an effective adjunct to drugs. Biofeedback may also help.

Arrhythmias
Palpitation, sinus tachycardia, and worsening of preexisting arrhythmias may all be produced by stress, probably via a sympathetic–parasympathetic imbalance.

Hypotension (Fainting)
Produced by fear, probably due to peripheral vasodilation and a decreased ventricular filling.

Congestive Heart Failure
Frequently develops after periods of stress. Anxiety tends to exacerbate the condition.

Raynaud's Disease
Can often be treated effectively with progressive relaxation or biofeedback.

Migraine
Attacks are often precipitated by stress. Treatment should include medication *and* biofeedback. Consider relaxation and psychotherapy also.

Respiratory

Bronchial Asthma
Occurs in people with a genetic predisposition and is made worse by acute and chronic stress. These patients are at risk for developing neurotic emotional reactions secondary to the respiratory disorder. There is good evidence that a wide variety of problem-solving and stress-reducing techniques (e.g., psychotherapy, family therapy, systematic desensitization, hypnosis, etc.) are effective at preventing attacks in many asthmatics and should be used in conjunction with medication.

Hay Fever
Patients have an increased sensitivity to their allergens when stressed but may also develop characteristic symptoms when no allergens can be identified.

Tuberculosis
Chronic stress often precedes development of the disease.

Hyperventilation Syndrome
A common ER presentation (see Chapter 8). Differentiate from panic disorder.

Gastrointestinal

Peptic Ulcer
Stress contributes to ulcer development, probably through its influence on the hypothalamic–pituitary–adrenal axis. The

chronically frustrated and angry patient with increased gastric HCL (hypersecretor) is at risk. Help the patient develop more stress-free life patterns. Relaxation therapy may be of value.

Ulcerative Colitis

Stressful emotional factors often precede disease development and can induce a relapse, but the mechanism is unclear. Non-confrontative supportive psychotherapy is indicated to help the patient adapt better to stress and to the illness and to help deal with the frequently associated anxiety and depression, but psychiatric care alone will not prevent relapses. Other intestinal conditions that are markedly influenced by psychosocial stress include *regional enteritis* (Crohn's disease) and *irritable bowel syndrome*. "Functional gastrointestinal disorders" may be associated with a history of physical and sexual abuse in women.

Obesity

Genetic and psychological factors interact. Improper conditioning around food habits, an overvaluation of food, and a negative body image (e.g., "fatso") are central. "Binge eaters" are particularly susceptible to stress. Supportive psychotherapy may be of some value, but behavior modification is most useful. Long-term success is limited; initial weight loss is frequent but relapses are very common. A change in lifestyle appears essential.

ANOREXIA NERVOSA (DSM-IV p. 544, 307.1), a disorder of profound weight loss without loss of appetite, usually develops in adolescence (F:M = 10–20:1), continues through the early 20s, and may end in death by starvation (5% over 5 years, 20% over 20 years). It is increasingly common in upper middle class females. These patients have a disturbed body image (feel fat despite dramatic visual evidence to the contrary) and are preoccupied with losing weight. They diet, exercise, and dangerously abuse diuretics and laxatives, even while family members and professionals attempt to stop them. Many anorexics (50% at some time during their course) also binge eat. Major depression, alcoholism, and anxiety disorders are likely to occur at some point (6).

A related condition, **BULIMIA NERVOSA** (DSM-IV p. 549, 307.51), is a chronic disorder characterized primarily by episodic eating binges in adolescent or early adult females

(F:M = 5–10:1) *of normal weight* who follow the gorging by self-induced vomiting (purging) or by inducing diarrhea with laxatives. These individuals are weight conscious and markedly depressed by their uncontrolled eating: Self-deprecation, major depression, and suicidal ruminations are common, as is substance abuse (25%). Endocrinologic, family history, and treatment findings are similar to those of anorexia, and some patients slip back and forth between the two conditions over time.

Anorexics often have hormone imbalances (e.g., amenorrhea), numerous signs of starvation (e.g., edema, bradycardia, and hypothermia), and associated features like ritual behavior (e.g., handwashing). The etiology is uncertain. In a few patients, anorexia is comorbid with avoidant and bulimia comorbid with borderline personality disorders. The families frequently have disturbed interpersonal patterns and an increased incidence of eating and affective disorders. Be certain to rule out a primary affective or schizophrenic disorder.

Treatment should be comprehensive: hospitalization for severe cases, individual *and* family therapy, behavior modification, and (maybe) antidepressants. In its early stages this condition is frequently overlooked, yet treatment can be life saving. Develop a high index of suspicion in thin young females. The 1° treatment goal for anorexics is to gain weight—all else is 2°. Anorexics, if they survive, tend to be chronically thin women. Bulimics, on the other hand, benefit most from the combination of outpatient cognitive-behavioral therapy *and* antidepressants (7) [e. g., fluoxetine, 20–60 mg/day (8)] (but relapses are frequent), whereas a few require antipsychotics. Short-term relapse rate (1–2 years) is close to 75%–80% but long-term (10 or more years) outcome of bulimics finds 50% or more symptom free and most of the rest with reduced symptoms.

Musculoskeletal

Rheumatoid Arthritis
Symptoms frequently worsen after emotional stress. Stress may be acting as an immunosuppressant. Depression is common in these patients. Psychotherapy is of little value in altering the course of the disease.

Tension Headaches
Caused by chronic muscular tension. Treat with mild analgesics and EMG feedback from the frontalis muscles or with relaxation techniques (often coupled with vigorous activity).

Spasmodic Torticollis
Exacerbated by stress. EMG biofeedback may be useful.

Fibromyalgia
A common (3–6,000,000 patients in United States) condition with widespread musculoskeletal aches, stiffness, and points of tenderness ("trigger points") that tends to respond to amitriptyline and multimodal psychotherapy, which includes cognitive-behavioral methods (9).

Low Back Pain
Treat multimodally.

Endocrine

Conditions that are exacerbated by stress include *hyperthyroidism* and *diabetes mellitus.* Acute and chronic stress may precipitate a thyroid crisis in genetically predisposed patients. Ketosis may be produced and maintained by stress in diabetics. Patients with either condition should receive psychotherapy if they have adopted self-destructive life habits and if they experience frequent relapses.

Genitourinary

Most gynecologic disorders reflect primarily an endocrine imbalance, but many of these conditions also can be influenced significantly by psychosocial stress. Psychosomatic influences are most evident for menstrual disorders (premenstrual tension, amenorrhea, oligomenorrhea), dyspareunia, frigidity, pseudocyesis, premature ejaculation, and impotence. Spontaneous abortion can be produced by major stress.

Chronic Pain

Chronic pain patients are common. The sources of their pain may or may not be identifiable. They often have been thoroughly evaluated medically, have experienced several unsuccessful surgical or medical procedures, and may or may not be currently iatrogenically addicted to analgesics (be wary of requests for Demerol, Percodan, Codeine, Darvon, Talwin, Valium, etc.). Nothing has helped, and the patients show evidence of depression, hopelessness, chronic anxiety, insomnia, chronic anger, interpersonal withdrawal, and/or somatic preoccupation. Their lives may be totally dominated by the pain.

Be certain that you are not dealing with conditions that mimic or complicate chronic pain (see Chapter 11):

1. Unrecognized treatable organic pathology;
2. Primary depression, anxiety disorder, or psychosis;
3. Unrecognized early delirium or dementia;
4. Drug addiction;
5. Conversion disorder;
6. Somatization disorder;
7. Pain disorder;
8. Hypochondriasis;
9. Histrionic personality disorder;
10. Malingering;
11. Compensation factors.

Always treat the chronic pain patient globally. Do not become overly concerned about whether the pain is "real" or "psychological"—it invariably will have elements of both, and treatments will be similar. Use whatever medical and surgical means are of value but *do not* stop there. Always explore and apply the multiplicity of available psychological treatments:

- First, detoxify the patient, if necessary.
- Take the patient and their pain seriously. Be interested, sympathetic, and hopeful. Be a continuing presence—see the patient regularly and do not abandon him.
- Help the patient identify and accept reasonable expectations. Encourage the patient to continue functioning—avoid hospitalization.
- Recognize that chronic administration of analgesics has limited usefulness and great risks yet can be done therapeutically. Attempt to use no drugs or nonaddicting drugs (e.g., antidepressants, major tranquilizers, antihistamines). Codeine is the preferable narcotic.

- Have the patient keep a pain diary. Work with the patient over time to help determine what variables improve or worsen the pain.
- Consider the variety of psychological techniques available (e.g., hypnosis, biofeedback, relaxation therapy, etc.). Encourage the patient to discover that he or she is "in control of his or her own pain." Use these methods within the context of a good therapeutic alliance. Consider family and group therapy. Help others in the patient's environment become more appropriately responsive to his or her pain.
- Consider some physical procedures (e.g., nerve block, dorsal column stimulators, acupuncture, rhizotomy, etc.). Avoid surgery if possible.
- Recognize that not all patients will improve markedly.

Other

Skin
A wide variety of psychosocial stressors can exacerbate certain skin conditions, including psoriasis, chronic urticaria, pruritus, and neurodermatitis (eczema). Research suggests that (a) warts (a contagious disease) may respond to hypnosis and (b) **TRICHOTILLOMANIA** (DSM-IV p. 621, 312.39; hair pulling, 1% or more of the population; F:M = 10^+ : 1) may respond to venlafaxine [37.5–450 mg/day (10)], fluoxetine, or clomipramine (related to OCD?).

Malignant Disease
Psychological stressors appear to influence the development (but perhaps not the course) of a malignancy. Isolation and depression are mild risk factors for cancer; their repair decreases that risk (11). This may be related to the effect of stress on the immune system. Much work remains to be done, yet there is some suggestion that psychological treatments (e.g., hypnosis) may play a future role in cancer treatment.

Hematologic
Stress may aid clotting among hemophiliacs. Changes in levels of various blood elements may occur in normal subjects under acute stress.

Accident Proneness
Some people are chronically at risk for accidental trauma due to psychological characteristics (e.g., impulsive, anxious, hostile).

Chronic Fatigue Syndrome
Despite extensive research, chronic fatigue syndrome (CFS) remains a puzzle (12). It is a chronic illness (greater than 6 months; 1% of the population) of unknown etiology (medical? psychological?) characterized by chronic fatigue (particularly postexercise), generalized pain and myalgia, fever and lymphadenopathy, insomnia and hypersomnia, and poor concentration and anterograde memory deficits. Depression is common (13), but antidepressants seldom produce marked improvement. Treatment is supportive, although cognitive-behavioral approaches seem to help (14). With luck, the future will bring clarity.

Seizures
Emotional stress can trigger seizures (both neurogenic and conversion). Psychotherapy and stress management is effective in helping to control seizure disorders, particularly in patients with partial seizures.

REFERENCES

1. Sapolsky RM. *Why zebras don't get ulcers*. New York: WH Freeman, 1998.
2. Wolman BB. *Psychosomatic disorders*. New York: Plenum, 1988.
3. Denollet J, Sys SU, Brutsaert DL. Personality and mortality after myocardial infarction. *Psychosomat Med* 1995;57:582–591.
4. Sifneos PE. Alexithymia: past and present. *Am J Psychiatry* 1996;153: 137–142.
5. Glassman AH, Shapiro PA. Depression and the course of coronary artery disease. *Am J Psychiatry* 1998;155:4–11.
6. Sullivan PF, Bulik CM, Fear JL, et al. Outcome of anorexia nervosa: a case-control study. *Am J Psychiatry* 1998;155:939–946.
7. Walsh BT, Wilson GT, Loeb KL, et al. Medication and psychotherapy in the treatment of bulimia nervosa. *Am J Psychiatry* 1997; 154:523–531.
8. Mayer LES, Walsh BT. The use of selective serotonin reuptake inhibitors in eating disorders. *J Clin Psychiatry* 1998;59:[Suppl 15]: 28–34.
9. Mason LW, Goolkasian P, McCain GA. Evaluation of a multimodal treatment program for fibromyalgia. *J Behav Med* 1998;21:163–178.

10. O'Sullivan RL, Keuthen NJ, Rodriguez D, et al. Venlafaxine treatment of trichotillomania: an open series of ten cases. *SNS Spectrum* 1998;3:56–63.

11. Spiegel D, Sephton SE, Terr AI, et al. Effects of psychosocial treatment in prolonging cancer survival may be mediated by neuroimmune pathways. *Ann N Y Acad Sci* 1998;840:674–683.

12. Johnson H. *Osler's web.* New York: Penguin Books, 1996.

13. Saltzstein BJ, Wyshak G, Hubbuch JT, et al. A naturalistic study of the chronic fatigue syndrome among women in primary care. *Gen Hosp Psychiatry* 1998;20:307–316.

14. Hotopf M, Wessely S. Chronic fatigue syndrome—mapping the interior. *Psychol Med* 1999;29:255–258.

Chapter 13

Psychiatric Symptoms of Nonpsychiatric Medication

Many medical patients develop psychiatric symptoms (1,2) due to treatment with medical drugs as a common side effect, as an idiosyncratic response, from administration of toxic amounts, or as the result of an untoward combination of drugs. Unrecognized, the responsible medications might be continued. Likely offenders are explored here.

ANTICONVULSANTS

Anticonvulsants as a group typically produce neuropsychiatric symptoms of various kinds when the dose exceeds the usual therapeutic range. Some, however, produce problems in a few patients even at normal doses.

- Carbamazepine: Sedation, irritability, and depression at the start of treatment.
- Phenacemide: Emotional lability, agitation, and confusion in a few.
- Phenobarbital: Normal blood levels (5–40 µg/mL) occasionally may produce irritability and mood disturbance, cognitive impairment, and/or confusion, whereas excessive dosage will produce sedation grading into ataxia and coma. Symptoms of withdrawal may occur if phenobarbital is stopped abruptly.
- Phenytoin: Irritability, nystagmus, tremor, and ataxia often begin at 20 µg/mL and worsen as the dose climbs.
- Primidone: Over 50% of patients experience sedation, irritability, weakness, and/or vertigo upon beginning the medication.

ANTI-INFLAMMATORY AGENTS

- Salicylates: In high doses can produce elation and euphoria grading into depression, confusion, and delirium.
- Nonsteroidal anti-inflammatory drugs (NSAIDs): About 10% of patients experience sedation and dizziness. In high doses, a few will produce anxiety, disorientation, and confusion.

HORMONES

- Exogenous thyroid: Excess can result in symptoms varying from restlessness and anxiety to a psychosis mimicking mania or acute schizophrenia. Inadequately treated patients may display symptoms of hypothyroidism [e.g., fatigue, depression, psychosis (*myxedema madness*)].
- Adrenal corticosteroids (e.g., cortisone, dexamethasone, prednisone): In addition to physical complications, excessive or chronic use can produce widely varying affective syndromes (e.g., euphoria and hypomania, fatigue, and *depression*) and/or degrees of a toxic psychosis. Steroid withdrawal can produce complaints of weakness and fatigue—suspect *pseudotumor cerebri* if coupled with headache, vomiting, and confusion.
- Estrogens: Restlessness, a sense of well-being, euphoria.
- Progesterones: May produce fatigue, irritability, tearfulness, and depression when given either alone or in combination as oral contraceptives (2%–30% of patients).
- Androgens: Restlessness, agitation, aggressiveness, euphoria.

ANTICHOLINERGICS

Anticholinergics are contained in numerous medications and can produce mild peripheral (dry mouth, hypotension) and central (lability, distractibility, restlessness) side effects. For a start, consider
- Antihistamines: Benadryl, Phenergan, Teldrin, Ornade, Dramamine.
- Antispasmodics: Pro-Banthine.
- Ophthalmic drops: *atropine,* homatropine, cyclopentolate.
- Antiparkinsonian drugs: Cogentin, Artane, Tremin, Kemadrin, Akineton.
- Others: Compoz, Excedrin PM, Sleep-Eze, Sominex, and others containing *scopolamine.*

At higher doses an *anticholinergic psychosis* (see Chapter 23) can be caused by a variety of these drugs. Treat psychosis with physostigmine 1–2 mg IM or slowly IV; repeat in 20 minutes if needed.

ANTIHYPERTENSIVES AND CARDIAC DRUGS

- Rauwolfia alkaloids (reserpine): Can cause nightmares, confusion, and profound depression in susceptible patients taking normal doses.
- Diuretics (thiazides, furosemide, ethacrynic acid): Fatigue.
- Methyldopa (Aldomet): Persistent lassitude, verbal memory impairment, depression with obtundation and confusion (on normal dosage).
- Guanethidine (Ismelin): Mild depression.
- Calcium channel blockers (flunarizine, cinnarizine; nifedipine, verapamil): Dizziness, lethargy, and euphoria are common with some medications; *depression* with others.
- Clonidine: Sedation, depression; antagonized by tricyclic antidepressants; hypomania on withdrawal sometimes.
- Propranolol (Inderal) and other beta-blockers: Fatigue, insomnia, nightmares, verbal memory impairment, and *depression;* hyperactivity, paranoia, rarely confusion, and a toxic psychosis.
- Digitalis and the cardiac glycosides: Fatigue, apathy, *depression,* and/or toxic delirium, particularly in the elderly.
- Antiarrhythmics (quinidine, procainamide, lidocaine): Mild confusion, mild-to-major delirium, occasionally depression.

SYMPATHOMIMETICS

Both catecholamine and noncatecholamine stimulants may produce restlessness, anxiety, fear and panic, weakness, dizziness, irritability, and insomnia in recommended dosages.

BROMIDE

Intoxication is rare; availability of bromide in medications has dropped to almost nothing. Chronic intoxication (weeks, months; "bromism") occurs very infrequently: symptoms range from mild disorientation to full toxic psychosis and dementia. Look for "classic" acneiform rash of face and hair roots (30% of patients).

LEVODOPA

The depression and apathy of Parkinson's disease may be relieved, but anxiety and agitation are produced frequently. About 15% of patients develop more serious psychiatric problems, including an acute organic brain syndrome with confusion or frank delirium, hypomania, acute psychosis, or major depression. Often hard to differentiate from the progression of the disease.

HYPOGLYCEMICS (INSULIN, TOLBUTAMIDE)

Symptoms of hypoglycemia occur, including restlessness, anxiety, and disorientation.

ANTIBIOTICS AND RELATED DRUGS

- Tetracyclines: Can produce emotional lability, depression, and confusion—from vitamin deficiencies secondary to alteration of colonic bacteria.
- Nalidixic acid and nitrofurantoin: Lethargy, rarely confusion.
- Isoniazid (INH): Euphoria, transient memory loss, agitation, psychotic reaction, paranoia, catatonic-like syndrome.
- Cycloserine: Lethargy and confusion, agitation, severe depression, psychosis, paranoid reactions.

ANTINEOPLASTICS

Acute organic brain syndromes and depression can be produced by a variety of these agents, either by a direct CNS effect or due to involvement of other systems (e.g., anemia).

REFERENCES

1. Brown TM, Stoudemire A. *Psychiatric side effects of prescription and over-the-counter medications.* Washington, DC: American Psychiatric Press, 1998.
2. Patten SB, Love EJ. Drug-induced depression. *Psychother Psychosom* 1997;66:63–73.

Chapter 14

Psychiatric Presentations of Medical Disease

Physical and psychiatric illnesses are closely interwoven (1). Both medical and psychiatric physicians should appreciate this interrelationship.

- 60% of patients needing mental health care are being treated by medical physicians.
- 50%–80% of the patients treated in medical clinics have a diagnosable psychiatric illness, and 10%–20% of medical patients suffer primarily from an emotional disorder.
- 50% of patients in psychiatric clinic populations have undiagnosed medical conditions.
- 10% of self-referred psychiatric patients have symptoms solely due to a medical illness.

Always evaluate psychiatric patients medically. Be particularly alert to patients presenting with depression, confusion, memory loss, anxiety, personality changes, psychosis of rapid onset, visual hallucinations, and illusions. Always be suspicious of symptoms of sudden onset in a patient, particularly one over 35 years old, who previously had been problem free. Recognize that patients (or their physicians) often can identify a "precipitating event" for even the most organic of psychiatric conditions—do not be fooled.

Always consider psychiatric possibilities for physical symptoms in medical patients. Take a good history, including past emotional problems. Why is the patient coming for help now?

PSYCHIATRIC SYMPTOMS

There are only a few typical psychiatric presentations and many different medical illnesses that can cause them. Some of the most common associations are listed below, although almost any physical condition can contribute to symptom production (Table 14.1).

MEDICAL DISEASES

No medical illness produces pathognomonic psychiatric symptoms, yet each has a typical *range* of presentations. Some of the most char-

TABLE 14.1   Common Associations for Psychiatric Symptoms

Presentation	Disease
Anxiety	Hyperthyroidism
	Hypoglycemia
	Pneumonia
	Acute intermittent porphyria
	Pheochromocytoma
	Mitral valve prolapse
	Angina pectoris
	Cardiac arrhythmias
	Hyper- and hypoparathyroidism
	Hypothyroidism
	Cushing's disease
	Menstrual irregularities
Depression	Hypothyroidism
	Debilitating disease
	Pneumonia, other infections
	Cushing's disease
	Addison's disease
	Pancreatic carcinoma
	Intracranial tumors
	Pernicious anemia
	Hyper- and hypoparathyroidism
Confusion, memory loss	Numerous medical conditions (see Chapters 5 and 6)
Mixed psychotic-hysterical symptoms	MS
	Wilson's disease
	SLE
	Intracranial tumors
	Hyperthyroidism
	Psychomotor epilepsy
	General paresis
	Huntington's chorea
	Metachromatic leukodystrophy
	Porphyria

acteristic are listed below, but more comprehensive sources are available. In many of these diseases, the patient develops psychiatric pathology before any medical signs or symptoms are noticed.

Cardiovascular Disease

Serious heart problems *very* commonly produce psychiatric symptoms, particularly in the elderly (2). The most common heart-related symptom is probably *depression,* regardless of whether the medical situation is CHF, survival after an MI, or postcardiotomy recovery. Also, heart patients who develop depression are at markedly increased risk for further heart problems, making treatment of the depression mandatory; SSRIs are currently the medications of choice (3). In addition to depression, serious heart disease increases the incidence of apathy, disinhibition, and cognitive impairment (4). Finally, a well-recognized syndrome, **postcardiotomy delirium**, occurs in *one third* of patients after open heart surgery and is characterized by symptoms that range from mild disorientation through hallucinations and paranoid delusions (5).

Endocrine

- Hyperthyroidism—anxiety (75%–80% meet criteria for GAD at some point), restlessness, emotional lability, weight loss, sweating, fine tremor, atypical depression with confusion in older patients.
- Hypothyroidism—depression (approximately one third of patients), fatigue, apathy, occasionally anxiety and psychosis ("myxedema madness"), dry skin, EEG slowing, cold intolerance, and persistent cognitive defects [even after return to normal hormone levels (6)].
- Hyperparathyroidism (7)—anxiety and irritability; depression, apathy, and fatigue; confusion and delirium; abdominal and bone pain, kidney stones, duodenal ulcer. Symptoms progress to psychosis and coma as the serum calcium levels rise.
- Hypoparathyroidism—similar to hyperparathyroidism but with anxiety and emotional lability more common; seizures, tetany.
- Hypoadrenalism (Addison's disease)—fatigue, apathy, depression, weakness, occasional confusion.
- Pheochromocytoma—anxiety, restlessness, apprehension and panic, flushing, headaches; all during attacks.

- Hypoglycemia—symptoms vary with blood sugar; episodic anxiety, tremor, sweating, personality changes, bizarre behavior.
- Diabetes mellitus—depression, apathy, confusion, intellectual dullness.
- Premenstrual syndrome (PMS)—as many as 25% of women develop significant physical/psychological discomfort during the 4–5 days before menses, ending shortly after flow begins. Common symptoms include irritability, tension, tearfulness, moderate depression, a sense of bloating, swelling of the extremities, and headaches, but may include more severe symptoms such as profound depression, aggressiveness, and even psychosis. The etiology is unknown but may be related to hormonal imbalance: possibly prolactin, estrogen, or prostaglandins. Women with a preexisting mood disorder may be at risk for problems. No treatment is certain, but progestogenic oral contraceptives, bromocriptine, Li, and/or psychotherapy may help.

Infections

Depression, anxiety, OBS, and acute psychosis all can occur due to a variety of infectious processes, depending on the patient's sensitivity, age and physical condition, the site of the infection, and the agent. Particularly common are symptoms with pneumonia (particularly delirium with bacterial and depression with viral), infectious mononucleosis (anxiety and psychosis may be the first symptoms; depression is commonly late), viral hepatitis (the posthepatitic syndrome: weakness, irritability, lethargy, depression), syphilis (general paresis), and TB. The reverse may also be true; psychiatric disorders such as depression may increase the risk for developing infections [e.g., herpes simplex virus (8)].

Other

- Acute intermittent porphyria (9)—15% of cases present first with psychiatric symptoms: anxiety, irritability, emotional outbursts, depression, acute psychosis; abdominal pain, peripheral neuropathies and bulbar palsies, vomiting and constipation.
- Hepatolenticular degeneration (Wilson's disease)—May present with a labile mood, explosive outbursts, and psychotic behavior in a young man before the development of cirrho-

sis, portal hypertension, rigidity, Kayser-Fleischer rings, and dementia.

- Pellagra—*Dementia, diarrhea,* and *dermatitis;* also depression, personality changes, and a confusional psychosis.
- Systematic lupus erythematosus (SLE)—Patient may present with confusion, an affective state, and psychotic behavior before physical signs appear.
- Pernicious anemia—Depression and fatigue but also an organic psychosis. Look at blood for characteristic megaloblastic anemia.
- Pancreatic carcinoma—Severe depression in 40% or more of patients. Also depression with CA of lung and brain.
- Prolapse of the mitral valve—Associated with generalized anxiety disorder, panic disorder, and agoraphobia with panic attacks, but the significance of the association is not known.
- Chronic obstructive pulmonary disease (COPD)—anxiety, depression, and mild to moderate organicity are common.
- Irritable bowel syndrome (10)—GI pain, distention, and gas; *also* psychiatric symptoms of autonomic arousal such as anxiety, panic, weakness, fatigue, headaches, tremor, insomnia, etc. (Is this fundamentally a psychiatric illness?)

REFERENCES

1. Lishman WA. *Organic psychiatry,* 3rd ed. Oxford: Blackwell Publishers, 1998.
2. Musselman DL, Evans DL, Nemeroff CB. The relationship of depression to cardiovascular disease: epidemiology, biology, and treatment. *Arch Gen Psychiatry* 1998;7:580–592.
3. Shapiro PA, Lidagoster L, Glassman AH. Depression and heart disease. *Psychiatric Ann* 1997;27:347–352.
4. Reich P, Regestein QR, Murawski BJ, et al. Unrecognized organic mental disorders in survivors of cardiac arrest. *Am J Psychiatry* 1983; 140:1194–1197.
5. Smith LW, Dimsdale JE. Postcardiotomy delirium: conclusions after 25 years? *Am J Psychiatry* 1989;146:452–458.
6. Leentjens AFG, Kappers EJ. Persistent cognitive defects after corrected hypothyroidism. *Psychopathology* 1995;28:235–237.
7. Borer MS, Bhanot VK. Hyperparathyroidism: neuropsychiatric manifestations. *Psychosomatics* 1985;26:597–601.
8. Zorrilla EP, McKay JR, Luborsky L, et al. Relation of stressors and depressive symptoms to clinical progression of viral illness. *Am J Psychiatry* 1996;153:626–635.

9. Tishler PV, Woodward B, O'Connor J, et al. High prevalence of intermittent acute porphyria in a psychiatric patient population. *Am J Psychiatry* 1985;142:1430–1436.

10. Gaynes BN, Drossman DA. The role of the mental health professional in the assessment and management of irritable bowel syndrome. *CNS Spectrums* 1999;4:19–30.

Chapter 15

Psychiatric Presentations of Neurologic Disease

Many psychiatric symptoms caused by various neurologic diseases (e.g., CNS tumor, trauma, seizure, infection) can be correlated directly to the CNS site involved.

FRONTAL LOBES

In prefrontal damage, the *frontal lobe syndrome* occurs with unilateral or bilateral damage (personality changes, irritability, euphoria, apathy, pseudodepression, impulsivity, social inappropriateness). Do not mistake for depression or mania. Intelligence is usually unimpaired in unilateral damage, although memory can be affected. Symptoms are milder if only one side is involved. If the premotor area is involved (on the left), there may also be apraxia of the left hand and Broca's (expressive) aphasia. Do not confuse with psychosis.

TEMPORAL LOBES

Stimulation or lesions may produce visual and olfactory hallucinations, noncomplex auditory hallucinations, and aggressive psychotic behavior. Dominant lobe lesion may produce agnosia for sounds, intonations, and music. Bilateral lesions may produce the amnestic disorder of Korsakoff and the Kluver-Bucy syndrome (placidity and hypersexuality).

PARIETAL LOBES

Dominant lobe lesions may produce language difficulties (e.g., inability to express or understand spoken words, perform simple tasks, read and/or write), tactile agnosia, apraxia, and intellectual deterioration. Nondominant lobe lesions may produce anosognosia.

OCCIPITAL LOBES

Some lesions produce crude flashing visual illusions and hallucinations.

LIMBIC SYSTEM

Effects are diverse but usually involve primitive and emotional behavior (e.g., emotional lability, fear, rage, impulsivity, depression, memory loss). Also, amnestic syndrome is seen when mammillary bodies are involved (Korsakoff's syndrome).

NEUROLOGIC DISEASES

Neurologic disorders can produce a variety of psychiatric symptoms. Consult a comprehensive source for detailed descriptions of specific conditions. Some major diseases are presented below.

- *Parkinson's disease* (1)—Frequently accompanied by apathy and depression (40%+), dementia (40%), and anxiety (40%).
- *Huntington's chorea*—May present first with psychiatric symptoms (e.g., emotional lability, impulsiveness, depression, hallucinations, delusions). Do not mistake for schizophrenia, major depression, or mania. Look for family history, movement disorder, and dementia.
- *Multiple sclerosis* (MS)—Early psychiatric symptoms are common, particularly *emotional lability,* euphoria, transient psychotic episodes, *depression* (2), and a "hysterical" presentation.
- *Intracranial tumors*—50% of patients develop psychiatric symptoms, and occasionally they may be the presenting symptoms. Pattern is site related, although there is usually a degree of generalized organicity. Early personality changes are often subtle (e.g., "He's not the same person any more"). Aphasias due to tumor (or any other cause) may mimic psychotic language disorders; there are qualitative differences between these two types of speech.

- *Head trauma* (3)—A postconcussion syndrome: includes irritability, emotional lability, and personality changes. Depression and mania may occur. Results can be long lasting.
- *CNS infection*—Typically presents with OBS (usually irritability and restlessness initially). General paresis (CNS syphilis) (4,5) usually presents as a gradually developing dementia but can produce a variety of confusing symptoms (e.g., may mimic schizophrenia, mania, depression, somatization disorder).
- *Stroke—Poststroke depression* is common (50% or more of patients) but the type of mood disorder tends to vary with the anatomic location of the damage (*very* uncertain as yet) (6): major depression (L-frontal; R-parietal); dysthymia (L- and R-posterior); unnatural cheerfulness, anxiety, and anhedonia (R-frontal); and mania (R-basotemporal). Major depression lasts for 9–12 months and responds to antidepressants or ECT. This localization work is poorly refined as yet.
- AIDS (7)—Some combination of apathy and depression, anxiety and agitation, and denial occur in many AIDS patients and requires therapy. Minor memory, language, and concentration abnormalities develop early in many; 50% or more develop serious neurologic complications later that often grade into delirium and dementia.
- **TOURETTE'S DISORDER** (DSM-IV p. 103, 307.23)—This neuropsychiatric syndrome of uncertain etiology usually develops in latency or early adolescence with the onset of one or more poorly controlled symptoms, including head or extremity tics, eyeblinks, and the spasmodic production of coughs or grunts that occasionally can include verbal obscenities (coprolalia). It is often severe and lifelong, occurs (along with other tic phenomena) with increased incidence in families, appears to have a major genetic component, and is associated (genetically?) with OCD and chronic tics (8) and also possibly with hyperactivity (ADHD) and learning disorders in family members. All symptoms are worsened by stress and may be improved by psychotherapy, but primary treatment is pharmacologic: haloperidol (past mainstay; 60%–70% of patients improve; 2–12 mg/day) but consider clonidine (0.1–0.5 mg/day; up to 50% respond), pimozide (9) (2–12 mg/day), risperidone (10), and clonazepam. Stimulant medication can precipitate or worsen Tourette symptoms but can also help, so use cautiously, if at all.

REFERENCES

1. Stacy M. Recognizing and treating nonmotor disorders associated with Parkinson's disease. *CNS Spectrums* 1998;3:41–45.
2. Schubert DSP, Foliart RH. Increased depression in multiple sclerosis patients. *Psychosomatics* 1993;34:124–130.
3. Mendel S, Sataloff RT, Schapiro SR. *Minor head trauma*. New York: Springer-Verlag, 1993.
4. Rundell JR, Wise MG. Neurosyphilis: a psychiatric perspective. *Psychosomatics* 1985;26:287–295.
5. Simon RP. Neurosyphilis. *Arch Neurol* 1985;42:606–613.
6. Singh A, Herrmann N, Black SE. The importance of lesion location in poststroke depression: a critical review. *Can J Psychiatry* 1998; 43:921–927.
7. Maj M, Satz P, Jonssen R, et al. WHO neuropsychiatric AIDS study: neuropsychological and neurological findings. *Arch Gen Psychiatry* 1994;51:51–61.
8. Alsobrook JP. The genetics of Tourette syndrome. *CNS Spectrum* 1999;4:34–53.
9. Sallee FR, Nesbitt L, Jackson C, et al. Relative efficacy of haloperidol and pimozide in children and adolescents with Tourette's disorder. *Am J Psychiatry* 1997;154:1057–1062.
10. Bruun RD, Budman CL. Risperidone as a treatment for Tourette's syndrome. *J Clin Psychiatry* 1996;57:29–31.

Chapter 16

Psychiatry of Alcohol

Alcohol is *the* major substance of abuse. About 68% of Americans drink, 12% are heavy drinkers (men 2:1), 10 million have alcohol abuse problems, the lifetime risk for alcoholism is 10%–14%, and 50% of homicides and automobile deaths are alcohol related. Certain populations are at risk (e.g., elderly urban blacks, urban Indians, bartenders, musicians). Finally, mixed abuse of alcohol and other drugs is extremely common.

CLASSIFICATION

Normal (recreational) drinking grades into pathologic use. **ALCOHOL ABUSE** (DSM-IV p. 196, 305.00) exists if there is clearly recurrent (not continuous) impaired social and occupational functioning due to alcohol use over a 1-year period. Individual patterns can vary from steady sporadic consumption to periodic binges. All demonstrate the inability to abstain from drinking or to stop drinking once started, despite an obvious downward spiral. Such drinking may result in depression and anxiety. Beginning often as evening and weekend drinking, the pattern usually becomes established by the late 20s in males (later in females) with gradual deterioration in some during their 30s and 40s. Spontaneous remissions can occur: In fact they are the norm, but they are temporary. *Blackouts* (anterograde amnesia for events that occurred during acute intoxication but while the patient was conscious and quite functional) often develop as drinking worsens.

If the patient also demonstrates tolerance (increased amounts needed to achieve effect), withdrawal, and/or compulsive and continuous use, he or she has **ALCOHOL DEPENDENCE (ALCOHOLISM)** (DSM-IV p. 195, 303.90). Cultural groups are differently affected (e.g., low among Jews and Orientals). All social strata are affected—fewer than 5% are "skid row" types. There is no "typical alcoholic personality." Alcoholism is comorbid with chronic anxiety disorders, mood disorders (particularly females), schizophrenia, dementia, and antisocial personality disorder; the presence of these conditions is often both (and/or) an effort to "self-medicate" with alcohol and the after effect of 1° alcoholism. Nevertheless, always rule out (or treat) these psychiatric disorders.

The etiology of alcoholism is unknown. Evidence for genetic biologic characteristics grows but is not without controversy (risk of developing alcoholism: one alcoholic parent = 4 times normal risk; both parents alcoholic = 60% risk) (1). Adoption studies indicate a genetic factor in some families: increased frequency of alcohol abuse and sociopathy among male relatives and possibly increased somatization among female relatives of alcoholics. Recent research identifies two groups of alcoholics (2):

Type 1—adult onset; steady, gradually escalating consumption; guilty, worried, rigid, perfectionistic, dependent, introverted; modest family history; both males and females; some recover completely; 75% of alcoholics.

Type 2—alcohol-seeking from adolescence and early adulthood; impulsive; distractible; risk-taking; antisocial characteristics with recklessness and aggression; *strong* family history; primarily males; very treatment resistant; 25% of all alcoholics.

Moreover, certain predictive biologic features of future alcoholism may be inherited by some first-degree relatives (particularly males) of alcoholics, e.g., a *resistance to intoxication* (the person who can "really hold his liquor" from an early age is at a *very* high risk to develop alcoholism), a subnormal cortisol rise after drinking (3), and a subnormal epinephrine release after stress (4). Alcohol stimulates the release of dopamine from the nucleus accumbens, producing euphoria. Over time the dopaminergic neurons atrophy and natural level of dopamine falls, producing malaise unless the level is stimulated by alcohol (i.e., very reinforcing). With abstinence, the alcoholic's dopamine level may take months or years to recover.

RECOGNIZING THE ALCOHOLIC

Clinical Markers

The *majority* of alcoholics function fairly well most of the time and go unrecognized by physicians until their social and occupational lives and their physical health have been significantly harmed. Early recognition is important. These patients frequently conceal alcohol use; keep a high index of suspicion if the predominant complaints include chronic anxiety and tension, insomnia, chronic depression, headaches, blackouts, nausea and vomiting, vague gastrointestinal problems, tachycardia, palpitations, and frequent falls or minor injuries. Ask about absenteeism, job loss, financial difficulties, and family trouble. Ask "Do you drink?" Be encouraging and nonjudgmental. Get drinking specifics (number of beers per day, oz/glass, drink alone?, etc). Interview relatives and friends, if possible.

Screening Tests

Use a brief screening questionnaire (but remember, patients often "fake good"). Two that are quick and reliable are the *SAAST* (Self-Administered Alcoholic Screening Test; accurate when computer scored; takes 10 minutes; also accurate when completed by a relative) (5) and the *CAGE* (consists of 4 "mnemonic" questions; two or more positive answers are suggestive of alcoholism) (6):

1. "Have you ever felt you should *C*ut down on your drinking?"
2. "Have people *A*nnoyed you by criticizing your drinking?"
3. "Have you ever felt bad or *G*uilty about your drinking?"
4. "Have you ever had a drink first thing in the morning to steady your nerves or get rid of a hangover (*E*ye opener)?"

There is also a subscale of the MMPI, the MacAndrew Scale (Mac), that consists of 49 MMPI items and provides a degree of reliability when coupled with the MMPI validity scales.

Biologic Markers

Chronic drinking frequently elevates serum gamma-glutamyl-transferase (GGT) and RBC MCV (together they identify 90% of alcoholics). These measures, coupled with evidence of more acute alcoholic insult (protein, Alk Phos, LDH, SGOT, SGPT, etc.), constitute a fairly reliable laboratory screen for alcoholism. A new blood test, carbohydrate-deficient transferrin (CDT), has demonstrated a sensitivity of 82% and specificity of 97% (7,8). It could be very useful but primarily when used with other tests because its sensitivity is very high and it is likely to pick up "normal heavy drinkers" (like college students).

CLINICAL PRESENTATIONS OF ALCOHOL SYNDROMES

When suspecting alcohol problems, always determine whether (a) the patient is *currently intoxicated* and (b) the time since the patient's *last drink*.

Intoxication Syndromes

ALCOHOL INTOXICATION (DSM-IV p. 196, 303.00)
Alcohol is a CNS depressant that initially disinhibits and then depresses. Early intoxication includes liveliness, a sense of well-being, and a smell of alcohol on the breath (blood alcohol levels up to 100 mg/100 mL); grading into irritability, emotional lability, and incoordination (100–150 mg%); which grades into apathy, slurred speech, and ataxia (150–250 mg%); which can become *alcoholic coma* (above 250–400 mg%, an emergency—get blood alcohol level and check for presence of other drugs; treat with intubation, CPR, etc., if necessary). Blood alcohol levels vary with drinking history and thus are only approximate.

Acute intoxication can mimic schizophrenia, mania, depression, hysteria, etc., so delay detailed interview and final diagnosis until the patient is sober. Evaluate *carefully* for medical problems (see below)—differential includes hypoglycemia, CNS infection, and toxic psychosis of other etiology. Intoxicated patients may be uncooperative, assaultive, and dangerous—be civil, non-threatening, accepting, respectful, patient, but prepared with force. Attempt nonpharmacologic management (quiet room, support, coffee), but sedation may be necessary (e.g., diazepam 5–20 mg IM, erratically absorbed), but be cautious of oversedation. Decide if the patient just needs to "sleep it off," is at risk for withdrawal, or is becoming comatose. Should the patient go home with family, be observed overnight, be hospitalized, or go to jail? Be familiar with community resources.

Alcohol idiosyncratic intoxication or pathological intoxication is an unusual and controversial condition (not currently in DSM-IV) of marked aggressiveness and emotional lability, occasionally of psychotic proportions, that follows ingestion of small quantities of alcohol in an otherwise normal person. Etiology is unknown. Some patients retain this pattern for life. Episodes appear suddenly and may last for hours or a day or more, often with amnesia for the episode afterward. Sedate (benzodiazepines, Haldol) and control until sober. Rule out temporal lobe epilepsy. *Alcoholic paranoia* has a similar presentation but with strong paranoid delusions: it usually occurs in chronic alcoholics who are actively drinking.

Alcohol Withdrawal Syndromes

These may occur in heavy drinkers or alcoholics who stop drinking *or* who *just reduce* their consumption. Do not overlook them in the "closet" alcoholic (e.g., the businessman or housewife who temporarily abstains while in the hospital for other reasons). If the patient is withdrawing, delay final diagnostic conclusions.

ALCOHOL WITHDRAWAL (DSM-IV p. 197, 291.8)

Tremulousness, hyperreflexia, weakness, nausea and vomiting, "dry heaves," anxiety, insomnia and bad dreams, mild illusions and hallucinations, hypervigilance, paresthesias, numbness, tinnitus, and/or blurred vision begin during the first 12–18 hours of reduced drinking and lead to a vicious cycle of worsening agitation. There is no EEG slowing; instead, the waves are normal or fast. Debilitated medically ill patients are at risk. *Alcoholic convulsions* (generalized, self-limited, single, or in small groups) occur in some (<25%), usually in the first 2 days of withdrawal but sometimes later. If the seizure is focal, suspect CNS pathology (e.g., subdural).

ALCOHOL WITHDRAWAL DELIRIUM (DSM-IV p. 131, 291.0)

Alcohol withdrawal delirium [*delirium tremens* (DTs)] is a life-threatening delirium that follows worsening withdrawal and is characterized by disorientation, agitation, memory disturbances, hallucinations (usually visual but also tactile, auditory, vestibular, etc.), delusions, powerful autonomic discharge (hypertension, tachycardia, sweating), tremor, ataxia, and fever beginning 2–8 days after reduced drinking. Tremulousness and seizures can precede, and often are mistaken for, the much less common DTs. Malnourishment and medical illness increases the risk of delirium. Mortality rate is 10%–15% for the complete syndrome (often from secondary infection or acute heart failure). Perhaps 1%–3% of alcoholics ever experience DTs.

ALCOHOL-INDUCED PSYCHOTIC DISORDER, WITH HALLUCINATIONS (DSM-IV p. 314, 291.3)

This disorder displays striking auditory hallucinations (voices, sounds) and mixed other withdrawal symptoms (mild tremor, anger, apprehension), but the patient typically has a *clear sensorium* and is *oriented*. It usually occurs in the first 3 days after cessation of drinking in patients who have had years of heavy drinking. Patients may be dangerous or self-destructive while hallucinating. It is usually self-limited (within 1 week), but occasional cases last for months or become chronic. Differential includes alcoholic paranoia and toxic psychosis (amphetamine, cocaine). Differentiation from paranoid schizophrenia is difficult in chronic cases (look for other signs of schizophrenia).

COMPLICATIONS OF CHRONIC ALCOHOLISM

Medical

Gastritis, gastric ulcer, diarrhea, anemia, hypertension, acute pancreatitis (after 10 or more years of drinking), cirrhosis (in less than 10% of alcoholics—alcohol plus poor diet), vitamin malabsorption (particularly A, B_{12}, thiamine, and folate), persistent impotence, insomnia, results of accidents. (***Note:*** Most alcoholics die 15 years early but not of these diseases, rather they die of heart disease and cancer.)

Neurologic

1. Peripheral neuropathy (vitamin B deficiencies);
2. Alcoholic cerebellar degeneration;
3. Central pontine myelinolysis;
4. Marchiafava-Bignami disease;

5. Cerebral atrophy;
6. Alcoholic myopathy and cardiomyopathy;
7. Wernicke's encephalopathy [the *triad:* confusion, ataxia, eye movement dysfunction (*vertical* and horizontal nystagmus and marked weakness of conjugate gaze and external rectus muscles)]—due to thiamine deficiency (give 50 mg IV and 50 mg IM, then 50 mg IM qd until patient is eating). An emergency—if treated early, it usually clears quickly and may prevent Korsakoff's syndrome.

Psychiatric

1. **ALCOHOL-INDUCED PERSISTING AMNESTIC DISORDER** (*Korsakoff's syndrome*) (DSM-IV p. 162, 291.1) is a profound short-term memory loss (thus anterograde amnesia but may also lose decades retrograde) with confabulation, which often abruptly follows untreated Wernicke's encephalopathy but may develop insidiously. Typically, events are remembered for several minutes and then are forgotten. Due to thiamine deficiency, lesions responsible for the anterograde amnesia are believed to be in the mammillary bodies, mammillo-thalamic tract, and anterior thalamus (previously thought to be in the dorsomedial thalamus). The retrograde amnesia and apathy found in many patients is believed to be due to diffuse frontal lobe damage. Treat as in Wernicke's disease. Impairment is often incapacitating and lifelong, yet 75% improve somewhat with time.
2. **ALCOHOL-INDUCED PERSISTING DEMENTIA** (DSM-IV p. 154, 291.2) refers to a dementia (i.e., all intellectual functions affected) that ranges from mild to severe and follows many years of alcohol abuse with no other obvious etiology. Few alcoholics are affected, and the predisposition is unknown.
3. Suicide—Alcohol is involved in many/the majority of suicides.
4. Drug abuse—Assume the serious drug abuser is a drinker, until proven otherwise.

Other

1. *Fetal alcohol syndrome* describes small, hyperactive, retarded children with variable anatomic abnormalities, including

ptosis, epicanthal folds, hypoplastic maxilla, cleft lip and palate, microcephaly, and hypospadias. Although not definite, it is thought to be due to a teratogenic effect on the fetus caused by alcohol consumed by the mother while pregnant. It is one of the most common causes of retardation (9).

TREATMENT OF WITHDRAWAL

Treatment varies with the severity of the symptoms (10). When in doubt, hospitalize temporarily; however, most patients manifesting mild withdrawal symptoms without medical complications can be treated in a supportive and *sober* environment, with daily clinic visits until stable and with good nutrition and occasionally little or no medication. The following apply to the more serious withdrawals.

1. Be clear and unambiguous. Identify yourself. Explain procedures. Place patient in a lighted room. Include family and familiar people. Use restraints if needed. Keep under *constant observation.*

2. *Carefully* evaluate (PE, chest x-ray, chemistry, electrolytes including calcium and magnesium, CBC, CT, occult blood in stool, occasionally an LP). Incidence of complicating disorders is high (e.g., pneumonia, TB, UTIs, hypoglycemia, diabetic ketoacidosis, anemia, shock, gastritis with hematemesis, acute hemorrhagic pancreatitis, cirrhosis and hepatic failure, meningitis). Be particularly careful to exclude (a) a *subdural hematoma* due to a fall and (b) withdrawal from other substances. Treat these conditions if present.

3. Use medication (11) to ensure sleep, prevent exhaustion, and reduce agitation. Use *benzodiazepines* to sedate until calm (but avoid oversedation) and control other symptoms and then taper over 4–8 days (i.e., decrease by approximately 20% of total first day's dose each day). If a delirium is present, it often resolves within 1 day. Next best alternative medication is probably carbamazepine (12) or depakote. Phenothiazines lower seizure threshold but may be useful with psychosis and extreme agitation.

   • *Tremulousness:* e.g., chlordiazepoxide 25–50 mg PO (or diazepam, 10–20 mg), every 4–6 hours until comfortable. Lorazepam (6–12 mg/day) or oxazepam may be better choices in patients with liver disease or confusion. Moderate levels of benzodiazepines may be all that is necessary in most mild to moderate withdrawals.

- *Delirium:* e.g., chlordiazepoxide 50–100 mg, PO or IM every hour until calm (able to stay in bed) and then q4 hrs. IM doses are often poorly absorbed—can lead to early undersedation, then cumulative oversedation. If patient is severe, give IV slowly. Benzodiazepines alone may not relieve delirium; consider low-dose haloperidol. Clonidine, a sympathetic inhibitor, may relieve sweating, tremor, and tachycardia but does not prevent DTs. Beta-blockers (e.g., atenolol, 50–100 mg/day) used with benzodiazepines may shorten the course.

4. If withdrawal seizures persist or a primary seizure disorder exists, consider 5–10 mg of diazepam slowly by IV or oral diphenylhydantoin, carbamazepine, or depakote combined with a benzodiazepine.

5. Give thiamine 100 mg IM and then 50 mg PO tid for 4 days. Also provide a high-carbohydrate diet and multivitamins daily (and for weeks/months).

6. Correct fluid and electrolyte imbalances, particularly hypokalemia (replace carefully over 24 hours or longer via IV) and significant hypomagnesemia (may exacerbate seizures—give magnesium sulfate 2–4 ml of 50% solution IM q6 hrs for 2 days).

7. Record pulse, BP, and temperature every half hour initially. Treat shock with fluids, whole blood, and vasopressors.

8. Check for and treat hypoglycemia, prolonged PT (give vitamin K 10 mg IM), and fever (aspirin, sponge baths—rule out superimposed infection).

9. Anxiety, irritability, depression, and insomnia may persist for weeks after the acute episode—a vulnerable period for the alcoholic. Even serious depression may spontaneously resolve after several weeks of sobriety; do not over (or under) treat. Antianxiety agents may be of use for several weeks but *do* discontinue.

TREATMENT OF ALCOHOLISM

Successful treatment of alcoholism is difficult but not hopeless. There is no definitive psychosocial treatment: Most alcoholics who

Drugs Used in Psychiatry

This guide contains color reproductions of some commonly prescribed major psychotherapeutic drugs. This guide mainly illustrates tablets and capsules. A † symbol preceding the name of a drug indicates that other doses are available. Check directly with the manufacturer. (*Although the photos are intended as accurate reproductions of the drug, this guide should be used only as a quick identification aid.*)

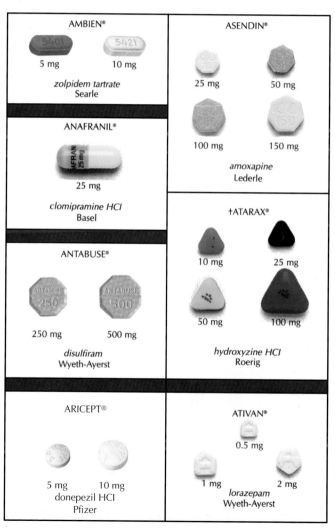

AMBIEN®	ASENDIN®
5 mg 10 mg	25 mg 50 mg
zolpidem tartrate Searle	100 mg 150 mg
ANAFRANIL®	amoxapine Lederle
25 mg	†ATARAX®
clomipramine HCl Basel	10 mg 25 mg
ANTABUSE®	50 mg 100 mg
250 mg 500 mg	hydroxyzine HCl Roerig
disulfiram Wyeth-Ayerst	
ARICEPT®	ATIVAN®
5 mg 10 mg donepezil HCl Pfizer	0.5 mg 1 mg 2 mg lorazepam Wyeth-Ayerst

Lippincott Williams & Wilkins©

BUSPAR®

5 mg   10 mg

buspirone HCl
Bristol-Myers Squibb

CELEXA®

20 mg   40 mg

citalopram
Forrest

†CLOZARIL®

100 mg

clozapine
Sandoz

†COGENTIN®

0.5 mg   1 mg   2 mg

benztropine mesylate
Merck & Co.

†COGNEX®

10 mg   20 mg   30 mg   40 mg

tacrine HCl
Parke-Davis

†COMPAZINE®

5 mg   10 mg   25 mg

prochlorperazine
SmithKline Beecham

†COMPAZINE® SPANSULE®

10 mg

15 mg

prochlorperazine
SmithKline Beecham

CYLERT®

18.75 mg
pemoline
Abbott

DALMANE®

15 mg

30 mg

flurazepam HCl
Roche

DEPAKENE®

250 mg

valproic acid
Abbott

Lippincott Williams & Wilkins©

DESOXYN®

5 mg

DESOXYN GRADUMET®

5 mg   10 mg   15 mg

methamphetamine HCl
Abbott

DEPAKOTE®

125 mg   250 mg

500 mg
divalproex sodium
Abbott

DESYREL®

50 mg   100 mg

trazodone HCl
Apothecon

†DESYREL® DIVIDOSE®

150 mg
trazodone HCl
Apothecon

† DEXEDRINE®

5 mg
dextroamphetamine
SmithKline Beecham

DORAL®

7.5 mg   15 mg

quazepam
Wallace Laboratories

†EFFEXOR®

37.5 mg   75 mg
venlafaxine HCl
Wyeth-Ayerst

EFFEXOR XR®

37.5 mg   75 mg   150 mg
venlafaxine HCl
Wyeth-Ayerst

†ELAVIL®

50 mg   75 mg

100 mg   150 mg
amitriptyline HCl
Stuart

Lippincott Williams & Wilkins©

†ELDEPRYL®

5 mg
selegiline HCl
Somerset Pharmaceuticals

HALDOL®

0.5 mg   1 mg   2 mg

5 mg   10 mg   20 mg

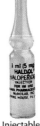

Concentrate   Injectable
2 mg per mL   5 mg/mL
                     (1 mL/ampul)

haloperidol
McNeil Pharmaceutical

†ENDEP®

50 mg   75 mg

100 mg   150 mg

amitriptyline HCl
Roche

†HALDOL® Decanoate

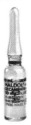

1 mL ampul
haloperidol
McNeil Pharmaceutical

†ESKALITH®

300 mg
lithium carbonate
SmithKline Beecham

HALCION®

0.125 mg   0.25 mg
triazolam
Upjohn

KEMADRIN®

5 mg
procyclidine HCl
Burroughs Wellcome

Lippincott Williams & Wilkins©

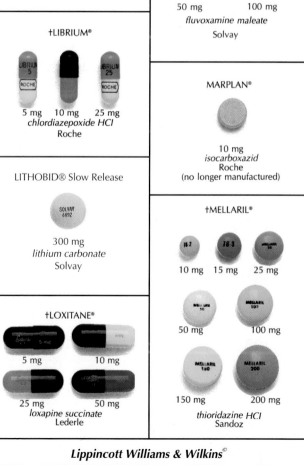

KLONOPIN®

0.5 mg   1 mg   2 mg
clonazepam
Roche

†LAMICTAL®

200 mg
iamotrigine
GlaxoWellcome

†LIBRIUM®

LIBRIUM 5   LIBRIUM 25
ROCHE   ROCHE

5 mg   10 mg   25 mg
chlordiazepoxide HCl
Roche

LITHOBID® Slow Release

SOLVAY
4492

300 mg
lithium carbonate
Solvay

†LOXITANE®

5 mg   10 mg

25 mg   50 mg
loxapine succinate
Lederle

LUDIOMIL®

25 mg   50 mg   75 mg
maprotiline HCl
Novartis

LUVOX®

SOLVAY 4205   SOLVAY 4210

50 mg   100 mg
fluvoxamine maleate
Solvay

MARPLAN®

10 mg
isocarboxazid
Roche
(no longer manufactured)

†MELLARIL®

10 mg   15 mg   25 mg

50 mg   100 mg

150 mg   200 mg
thioridazine HCl
Sandoz

Lippincott Williams & Wilkins©

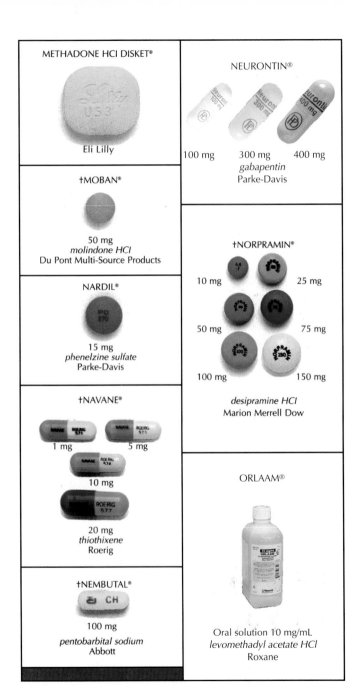

METHADONE HCI DISKET®

Eli Lilly

NEURONTIN®

100 mg   300 mg   400 mg
gabapentin
Parke-Davis

†MOBAN®

50 mg
molindone HCl
Du Pont Multi-Source Products

NARDIL®

15 mg
phenelzine sulfate
Parke-Davis

†NORPRAMIN®

10 mg   25 mg

50 mg   75 mg

100 mg   150 mg

desipramine HCl
Marion Merrell Dow

†NAVANE®

1 mg   5 mg

10 mg

20 mg
thiothixene
Roerig

ORLAAM®

†NEMBUTAL®

100 mg
pentobarbital sodium
Abbott

Oral solution 10 mg/mL
levomethadyl acetate HCl
Roxane

Lippincott Williams & Wilkins©

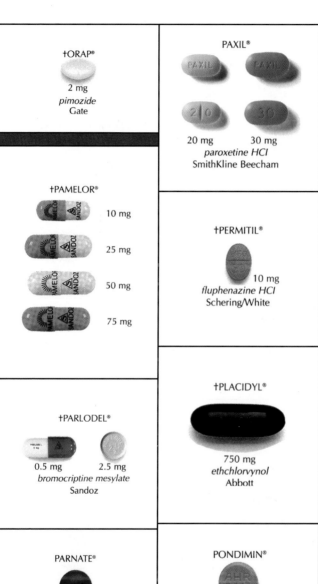

†ORAP®

2 mg
pimozide
Gate

PAXIL®

PAXIL   PAXIL

2|0   30

20 mg   30 mg
paroxetine HCl
SmithKline Beecham

†PAMELOR®

10 mg

25 mg

50 mg

75 mg

†PERMITIL®

10 mg
fluphenazine HCl
Schering/White

†PARLODEL®

0.5 mg   2.5 mg
bromocriptine mesylate
Sandoz

†PLACIDYL®

750 mg
ethchlorvynol
Abbott

PARNATE®

10 mg
tranylcypromine sulfate
SmithKline Beecham

PONDIMIN®

20 mg
fenfluramine HCl
A.H. Robins
(no longer manufactured)

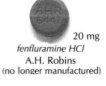

Lippincott Williams & Wilkins©

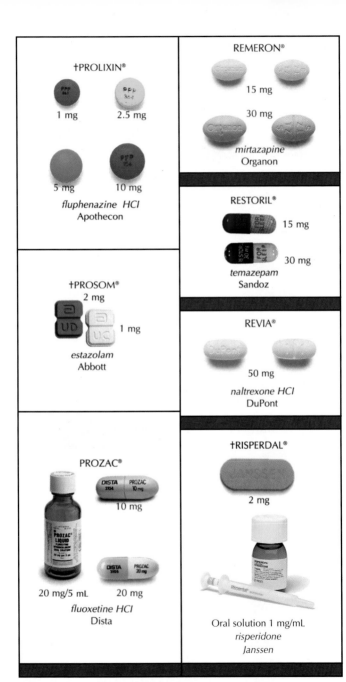

†PROLIXIN®

1 mg 2.5 mg

5 mg 10 mg

fluphenazine HCl
Apothecon

†PROSOM®
2 mg

1 mg

estazolam
Abbott

PROZAC®

DISTA PROZAC
3104 10 mg
10 mg

DISTA PROZAC
3105 20 mg
20 mg/5 mL 20 mg

fluoxetine HCl
Dista

REMERON®

15 mg

30 mg

mirtazapine
Organon

RESTORIL®

15 mg

30 mg

temazepam
Sandoz

REVIA®

50 mg

naltrexone HCl
DuPont

†RISPERDAL®

2 mg

Oral solution 1 mg/mL
risperidone
Janssen

Lippincott Williams & Wilkins©

RITALIN®

5 mg

10 mg

20 mg

methylphenidate HCl
Novartis

SERZONE®

100 mg

150 mg

200 mg

250 mg

nefazodone HCl
Bristol-Myers Squibb

†SERAX®

 10 mg

 15 mg

 30 mg

oxazepam
Wyeth-Ayerst

†SINEQUAN®

10 mg

25 mg

50 mg

75 mg
doxepin HCl
Roerig

†SERENTIL®

10 mg
mesoridazine besylate
Boehringer Ingelheim

†SPARINE®

25 mg

50 mg

100 mg
promazine HCl
Wyeth-Ayerst

SEROQUEL®

25 mg 100 mg 200 mg
quetiapine fumarate
Zeneca

Lippincott Williams & Wilkins©

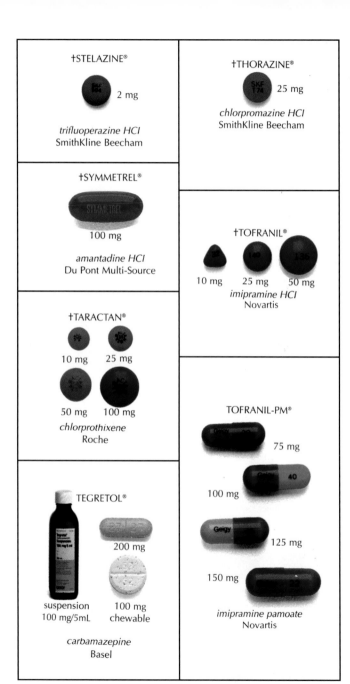

†STELAZINE®

2 mg

trifluoperazine HCl
SmithKline Beecham

†THORAZINE®

25 mg

chlorpromazine HCl
SmithKline Beecham

†SYMMETREL®

100 mg

amantadine HCl
Du Pont Multi-Source

†TOFRANIL®

10 mg   25 mg   50 mg
imipramine HCl
Novartis

†TARACTAN®

10 mg   25 mg

50 mg   100 mg

chlorprothixene
Roche

TOFRANIL-PM®

75 mg

100 mg   40

Geigy   125 mg

150 mg

imipramine pamoate
Novartis

TEGRETOL®

200 mg

100 mg
chewable

suspension
100 mg/5mL

carbamazepine
Basel

Lippincott Williams & Wilkins©

TOPAMAX®

25 mg   100 mg   200 mg

topiramate
Ortho-McNeil

†TRILAFON®

4 mg
perphenazine
Schering

†TRANXENE® T-TAB®
Tablets

7.5 mg
clorazepate dipotassium
Abbott

†VALIUM®

2 mg   5 mg   10 mg

diazepam
Roche

TRIAVIL®

2-10   2-25

4-10

4-25   4-50

perphenazine-amitriptyline HCl
Merck & Co.

†VISTARIL®

25 mg

50 mg

100 mg
hydroxyzine pamoate
Pfizer Laboratories

Lippincott Williams & Wilkins©

VIVACTIL®

5 mg   10 mg

protriptyline HCl
Merck & Co.

ZOLOFT®

100 mg   50 mg

sertraline HCl
Roerig

†WELLBUTRIN®

75 mg

100 mg
bupropion HCl
Burroughs Wellcome

ZYBAN®

ZYBAN
150

150 mg
bupropion HCl
GlaxoWellcome

†WELLBUTRIN SR®

100 mg
bupropion HCl
GlaxoWellcome

†XANAX®

0.25 mg   0.5 mg

1.0 mg   2.0 mg
alprazolam
Upjohn

ZYPREXA®

LILLY
4115

5 mg

LILLY
4116

7.5 mg

LILLY
4117

10 mg

olanzapine
Eli Lilly

Lippincott Williams & Wilkins©

become abstinent do so in addition to treatment, not because of it [see the classic *50-year* follow-up study of male alcoholics (13)].

1. Identify its presence. Get your facts straight (family drinking history, recent intake).
2. Develop a personal rapport with the patient—be warm and supportive but firm. Be open and matter-of-fact about the drinking but insist on abstinence. Remember, you cannot really evaluate/work with a patient unless he or she is abstinent—wait until the patient is sober before investing time in treatment. Encourage the patient to maintain employment and social involvement. Help develop coping skills. Although it may seem cruel, allow the patient to experience the "natural consequences" of his or her behavior, but use good judgment in doing so.
3. Treat all medical complications of drinking.
4. Treat any complicating primary psychiatric illness (e.g., schizophrenia, affective disorder, anxiety disorder). If the patient is likely to drink, recognize that tricyclics potentiate the CNS depressant effect of alcohol and that alcohol can promote lithium toxicity.
5. Enlist family members in treatment. Evaluate family's contribution to the problem. Consider family and/or marital therapy.
6. *Naltrexone* (14) (ReVia; 50 mg/day) is very promising (FDA approved) (15): It *decreases craving* (i.e., reduces the euphoria of alcohol and thus the drive to drink) in many alcoholics. Typically used for 3–6 months in conjunction with intensive psychosocial interventions; may be needed long-term if craving and relapse return. Another promising (but unavailable—soon perhaps) anticraving agent is *acamprosate* (16). Other (infrequently) effective drugs when used alone but better when used in special cases include lithium (with mania/depression), buspirone (in the anxious alcoholic), bromocriptine (possibly), and antidepressants (definitely should be used when the patient is also depressed).
7. Consider disulfiram (Antabuse; a "sensitizing" agent) use in cooperative but backsliding patients. It inhibits aldehyde dehydrogenase, leading to toxic acetaldehyde buildup 15–30 minutes after alcohol consumption, which leads to anxiety and apprehension, sweating, nausea and vomiting, tachycar-

dia, headache, and hypotension. Give 500 mg PO QD for 1 week and then maintain on 250 mg daily (range 125–500 mg). Carefully inform patient of the possible reactions. Effects last up to 2 weeks after last dose; however, not every patient shows an Antabuse reaction. Occasional adverse effects include sedation, a metallic taste, mild GI disturbances, mild ataxia, and a peripheral neuropathy. Question its use in thoroughly irresponsible patients; hepatotoxicity and toxic psychoses can occur and severe reactions (to a large alcohol challenge) can lead to shock and coma. Contraindicated in patients with unstable medical conditions or histories of psychosis, OBS, MI, or heart failure. The biggest problem with disulfiram: patients stop taking it so they can drink.

8. *Group therapy* appears to be the most effective psychotherapy technique. In most cases, work with or refer patients to a specialized multidisciplinary treatment team. Make referral personally, with the patient present. Alcoholics Anonymous (AA) can help some (although it has a very high initial drop-out rate)—encourage patients to give it a try. Alanon (spouses of alcoholics) is also useful. Hospitalize in an alcohol unit (milieu therapy) if even temporary sobriety cannot be achieved.

9. Be patient. Keep trying.

REFERENCES

1. Schuckit MA, Smith TL, Anthenelli R, et al. Clinical course of alcoholism in 636 male inpatients. *Am J Psychiatry* 1993;150:786–792.
2. Sigvardsson S, Bohman M, Cloninger CR. Replication of the Stockholm Adoption Study of Alcoholism. *Arch Gen Psychiatry* 1996;53: 681–687.
3. Schuckit MA, Gold E, Risch C. Plasma cortisol levels following ethanol in sons of alcoholics and controls. *Arch Gen Psychiatry* 1987; 44:942–945.
4. Swartz CM, Drews V, Cadoret R. Decreased epinephrine in familial alcoholism. *Arch Gen Psychiatry* 1987;44:938–941.
5. Davis LJ, Morse RM. Age and sex differences in the responses of alcoholics to the Self-Administered Alcoholic Screening Test. *J Clin Psychol* 1987;43:423–480.
6. Ewing JA. Detecting alcoholism. The CAGE questionnaire. *JAMA* 1984;252:1905.
7. Yeastedt J, LaGrange L, Anton RF. Female alcoholic outpatients and female college students: a correlational study of self-reported alcohol

consumption and carbohydrate-deficient transferrin levels. *J Stud Alcohol* 1998;59:555–559.

8. Wetterling T, Kanitz RD, Rumpf HJ, et al. Comparison of cage and mast with the alcohol markers CDT, gammaGT, ALAT, ASAT and MCV. *Alcohol* 1998;33:424–430.

9. Steinhausen HC, Spohr HL. Long-term outcome of children with fetal alcohol syndrome: psychopathology, behavior, and intelligence. *Alcohol Clin Exp Res* 1998;22:334–338.

10. Myrick H, Anton RF. Treatment of alcohol withdrawal. *Alcohol Health Res World* 1998;22:38–43.

11. Mayo-Smith MF. Pharmacological management of alcohol withdrawal: a meta-analysis and evidence-based practice guideline. *JAMA* 1997;278:144–151.

12. Malcolm R, Ballenger JC, Sturgis ET, et al. Double-blind controlled trial comparing carbamazepine to oxazepam treatment of alcohol withdrawal. *Am J Psychiatry* 1989;146:617–621.

13. Vaillant GE. *The natural history of alcoholism revisited.* Boston, MA: Harvard University Press, 1995.

14. O'Brien CP, Volpicelli LA, Volpicelli JR. Naltrexone in the treatment of alcoholism: a clinical review. *Alcohol* 1996;13:35–39.

15. Schaffer A, Naranjo CA. Recommended drug treatment strategies for the alcoholic patient. *Drugs* 1998;56:571–585.

16. Whitworth AB, Fischer F, Lesch OM, et al. Comparison of acamprosate and placebo in long-term treatment of alcohol dependence. *Lancet* 1996;347:1438–1442.

Chapter 17

Psychiatry of Drug Abuse

Drug abusers are common (6% lifetime prevalence in the U.S. as a whole, but pockets with much higher prevalence; M > F for all age groups), often unrecognized, and poorly understood. There is great variability in the degree of drug use from patient to patient (1); *multiple drug use* is common. *Abuse* occurs if the patient (A) uses drugs in a dangerous, self-defeating, self-destructive way; (B) has difficulty controlling use even though the use may be sporadic; and (C) has impaired social and/or occupational functioning because of that use, all within a 1-year period. Drug *dependence* requires the presence of tolerance, withdrawal, and/or continuous compulsive use over a 1-year period. Patients may be classified by the type of drug abused (see below) or by the pattern and reason for abuse. Some recognized patterns of use (abuse) include

- **Recreational use:** Patients take drugs "for fun" and are not physically or psychologically dependent on them. They may also take them just to be part of the group (e.g., adolescents) or because it is a countercultural requirement. This slowly may grade into compulsive use.
- **Iatrogenic addiction:** Patients addicted "by mistake." Patients (and physicians) may or may not recognize the addiction. Many of these patients are convinced that they must have the drug to function (e.g., to sleep, to interact with others) and may go to great lengths to talk their physician(s) into prescribing medication.
- **Chronic drug addiction:** These patients usually abuse "street" drugs (but not always, e.g., pain medications, seditive-

hypnotics). Many have underlying depressions. Many have antisocial personalities. Some take drugs to self-medicate a chronic psychiatric disorder (e.g., major depression, schizophrenia).

Drug abusers are not "all alike," but they do have many common features, including the frequent presence of marked depression and anxiety, increased dependency needs (often hidden), low self-esteem, a familial association (genetic?) with antisocial personality disorder and alcoholism, a dysfunctional family, and a chronic course resistant to treatment. Drug use to "self-medicate" specific psychiatric illnesses (anxiety, depression, panic disorder, schizophrenia) accounts for a modest amount of abuse. More commonly, however, it is the reverse: Chronic drug abuse produces emotional problems.

Treatment of chronic drug abusers is difficult; frequently an inpatient setting is required. Whether inpatient or outpatient, drug abusers should be treated firmly but with support and understanding. Set clear limits and stick to them. Deal with the patient only when he or she is not intoxicated (except for an acute crisis, of course). Be reasonably challenging. You will be tested and manipulated by many patients—do not respond with retribution. Follow many of the principles used in treating the alcoholic patient (see Chapter 16). Involve peers in a formal way (e.g., group therapy). The most common drugs of abuse, their clinical presentations, and treatment follow.

OPIOIDS

Drugs involved include
- Opium (principle active ingredient = morphine)
- Morphine
- Diacetylmorphine (heroin, horse, smack)
- Methadone
- Codeine
- Oxycodone (e.g., Percodan, in mixture)
- Hydromorphone (Dilaudid)
- Pentazocine (Talwin)
- Meperidine (Demerol)
- Propoxyphene (Darvon)
- Hydrocodone (Lortab, and others)

Some of these compounds are naturally occurring (opium and its constituents morphine and codeine), whereas others are semisynthetic or wholly synthetic. Some of these drugs have legitimate uses (e.g., morphine, meperidine), whereas others are solely substances of abuse (e.g., heroin). Most are obtained illegally "on the street" and are used primarily by a young or middle-aged lower socioeconomic population (although heroin is becoming "fashionable" among higher social classes currently), whereas others are abused more widely (e.g., Demerol, Dilaudid, and Percodan are commonly abused by professionals). Opioid drugs bind to *mu, kappa, delta,* and *lambda* **locus ceruleus** cell receptors (particularly **mu**) and inhibit norepinephrine release, producing the "high" of opioid abuse. After several weeks, the mu receptors have adjusted to the excess stimulus, and when the drug is stopped the "mu agonist withdrawal syndrome" or norepinephrine hyperactivity of the locus ceruleus begins, producing the withdrawal syndrome.

Typical routes of administration are IV (heroin, morphine, methadone—"mainlining"), SC (heroin, meperidine), nasally (heroin—"snorting"), orally (methadone, Percodan), and smoked (opium). It is frequently very difficult to determine the daily dose used because (a) the abuser often consciously over- or underestimates the dose and (b) the amount of active drug in a "bag" bought on the street is uncertain. A bag of heroin may be 95% adulterants (e.g., quinine, mannitol, lactose), although recently the purity of street heroin has increased (some bags being >50% heroin).

Abuse (**OPIOID ABUSE,** DSM-IV p. 249, 305.50) and dependency (**OPIOID DEPENDENCE,** DSM-IV p. 248, 304.00) are common in some populations, and the search for drugs or money for drugs accounts for most crime in some communities. Some people (less than 50%) are able to abuse opioids without becoming dependent (i.e., without progressing to tolerance and/or withdrawal), and they often use them recreationally without addiction. Those persons who become dependent represent a high-risk group. Recognize that we currently seem to be in an heroin epidemic similar to the "crack" epidemic of a decade ago: Inexpensive high-quality heroin is readily available and seems targeted at youth (e.g., heroin use has doubled among eighth graders over the past decade).

- 1% or more of all heroin addicts in the United States die each year; 25% die within 10–20 years from beginning their habit. Most common cause is an inadvertently fatal OD (e.g., an addict using "bags" of 5% heroin accidentally buys a supply containing 15% heroin). Also common is death during violent crime or, increasingly, AIDS.
- 25% or more of addicts have a personality disorder, usually of the antisocial type. They also have a high incidence of depression and anxiety. Suicide rate is elevated.
- Heroin addicts are at markedly increased risk (dirty needles, poor nutrition, etc.) for developing certain medical illnesses such as HIV/AIDS, but also:
  serum or infectious hepatitis
  SBE
  pneumonia, TB; pulmonary edema, embolus, abscess
  cellulitis, thrombophlebitis, septicemia
  UTIs, glomerulonephritis, nephrosis
  STDs
  Needle "tracts" on the arms (and legs).

Always carefully evaluate hospitalized addicts medically. Recognize that the analgesic properties of opioids may obscure acute medical problems. After several weeks of use, addicts lose the rush and are left with chronic anxiety and dysphoria. Still, the craving and hope for euphoria is so strong, and withdrawal so unpleasant, that they continue to abuse. Most addicts "grow out of" their habit over the years (or die); thus, there are relatively few old abusers.

Treatment of the opioid addict usually means treatment of the acute episodes (e.g., intoxication and withdrawal; see below). "Cure" of the addiction does occur in some well-motivated patients [and is particularly possible in new young (e.g., teen) addicts], yet most addicts continue their abuse over many years. The two major forms of *maintenance* treatment (both with controversial results) are

1. Agonist maintenance:(a) Patients are maintained as outpatients on daily doses of ***methadone*** of 40–120 mg. This level controls the craving for (and eliminates the euphoria from) heroin. The patient can then develop some skills, hold a job, go to school, etc. Psychotherapy can help some, but treatment demands careful limit setting (20%–50% of

patients abuse cocaine and/or alcohol while taking methadone). Moderately motivated patients *may* succeed by this route. Patients remain on methadone 1–20 or more years (or life). (b) **LAAM** (levo-alpha-acetylmethadol; ORLAAM, an oral solution), a chemical congener of methadone, has recently found use as a long-acting replacement for methadone (80 mg, 3 times/week) (2). Unfortunately, many of these patients as well continue to abuse other drugs while taking LAAM (cocaine and "crack" are common). (c) A new long-acting, injectable, partial opioid agonist, *buprenorphine* (Buprenex), appears safe [although there is some concern when given with benzodiazepines—deaths have occurred (3)], is given daily, and, perhaps most importantly, appears to decrease the patient's craving for cocaine as well (4).

2. Residential, drug-free, self-help programs: Patients (usually highly motivated) stay 1–2 years (or more) in a close "therapeutic community" that insists on the drug-free state and on personal responsibility. Confrontation and behavior modification are frequently used. "Poor" candidates usually drop out. Similar outpatient programs are common.

The two major features of illicit opioid use that bring patients to medical attention are intoxication (and overdosage) and withdrawal. **OPIOID INTOXICATION** (DSM-IV p. 249, 292.89) develops rapidly after an IV dose (1–5 minutes). The time course of intoxication varies with the drug used (Table 17.1). The abstinence syndrome begins after this period of time in the dependent patient. It is because of these kinetics that many heroin addicts "shoot up" 3–4 times/day, or more. **Intoxication symptoms** are similar for most narcotics.

Psychological symptoms: a rush immediately follows IV administration (described as a "whole body orgasm" with the focus in the abdomen). This is accompanied by euphoria and a sense of well-being or dysphoria (usually anxiety and fear), a drowsiness and "nodding off," apathy, psychomotor retardation, and difficulty concentrating.

TABLE 17.1   Time Course for Opioid Intoxication

Drug	Duration of action (hr)
Heroin	4–6
Methadone	12–24
Meperidine	2–4

Physical symptoms: miosis (*pupillary constriction*), slurred speech, respiratory depression, hypotension, hypothermia, bradycardia, constipation, and nausea and vomiting. Skin ulcers are common with meperidine injection. Seizures may occur in the patient tolerant to meperidine.

An OD (either accidental or intentional) is a medical emergency; these patients may die of respiratory depression and pulmonary edema. Look for needle tracts and pinpoint pupils in the unconscious patient but recognize that if the patient already has experienced significant CNS anoxia, the pupils may be dilated. Seizures occasionally occur (particularly with meperidine).

Treat the OD with intensive medical care (ICU) and the narcotic antagonist naloxone (Narcan). Give 0.4 mg IV and repeat 5 times at 3-minute intervals. Expect a rapid response (i.e., clearing in 1–2 minutes), and if this does not occur after four doses, suspect another etiology for the coma. If the patient improves, continue monitoring. The patient probably will need additional doses of naloxone because it has a much shorter half-life than either heroin or methadone. Excessive naloxone may throw a dependent patient directly from coma into withdrawal—do not be confused. Multiple drugs may have been taken—be alert to the possibility of a more slowly developing coma from a second agent. Of course, get a STAT urine drug screen.

Despite its reputation as a dramatic and traumatic withdrawal syndrome, **OPIOID WITHDRAWAL** (DSM-IV p. 251, 392.0) is uncomfortable but usually not life-threatening in healthy young adults and is not as dangerous or as difficult to manage as the withdrawal from sedative-hypnotic drugs. **Withdrawal symptoms** are similar for each of the narcotics, but the time course varies (dependent partly on the "size of the habit") (Table 17.2).

TABLE 17.2   Time Course for Opioid Withdrawal

Drug	Time after last dose that symptoms began (hr)	Symptoms peak	Symptoms disappear (days)
Heroin	4–8	1–3 days	7–10
Methadone	12–48	4–6 days	10–21
Meperidine	2–4	8–12 hr	4–5

Psychological symptoms: early on there is often intense drug crav-ing followed by severe anxiety, restlessness, irritability, insomnia, and decreased appetite. In this state, the hospitalized patient is fre-quently extremely demanding and manipulative.

Physical symptoms: yawning, diaphoresis, tearing, rhinorrhea, *pupillary dilation, piloerection* (hard to "fake" so look for it), muscle twitching, and hot flashes. Later there is nausea and vomiting, fever, hypertension, tachycardia, tachypnea, diarrhea, and abdom-inal cramps. Seizures occur with meperidine withdrawal.

Newborn addicts: infants born to addicted mothers, including those on methadone maintenance, often experience an abstinence syndrome, including a high-pitched cry, irritability, tremor, fever, decreased food intake, vomiting, yawning, and hyperbilirubinemia.

Be aware, successful withdrawal is only the beginning of the treatment of opiate dependence. **Withdraw** opioid addicts gradu-ally by using oral methadone (chosen because of long half-life) to lessen the symptom severity. After a complete history and physical (including urine screen for opioids and other drugs), wait for signs of withdrawal and then give methadone 5 mg PO. Establish the sta-bilization dose over the first 1–2 days by adding 5–10 mg of methadone on a qid schedule as the patient continues to show *signs* of abstinence (recognize that some patients will vigorously demand more drugs even while they are sedated by their current dose). Once stabilized, give the methadone on a QD or bid schedule and reduce the total daily amount by 5 mg/day (or 10%–20% of the sta-bilization dose; more slowly with outpatients). Most withdrawals from heroin addiction take 7–10 days, and methadone addiction withdrawals should be done more slowly (e.g., 2–3 weeks).

An alternate method of opiate withdrawal is to use *clonidine* (Catapres), which reduces withdrawal symptoms by stimulating the α_2-adrenergic receptors on the locus ceruleus (0.1 mg q4–6 hours until stable to maximum of 1.2 mg/day and then taper 0.1–0.2 mg/day) (5). (Withdraw patients from Talwin using decreasing doses of Talwin.) Many patients who become free of their drug find the craving irresistible and need to be maintained on methadone to stay "clean." Naltrexone seems to block the euphoric effects of the opioids (50 mg daily), as it does with alco-hol, but is of uncertain utility due to noncompliance.

If a patient is withdrawing from both opioids and sedative-hypnotics (not uncommon), concentrate on a safe sedative-hypnotic withdrawal by maintaining the patient on 10–30 mg of methadone until the first withdrawal has been completed.

SEDATIVE-HYPNOTICS

- **Benzodiazepines:** alprazolam (Xanax), chlordiazepoxide (Librium), clonazepam (Klonopin), clorazepate (Tranxene), diazepam (Valium), estazolam (ProSom), flurazepam (Dalmane), halazepam (Paxipam), lorazepam (Ativan), oxazepam (Serax), prazepam (Centrax), quazepam (Doral), temazepam (Restoril), triazolam (Halcion)
- **GABA$_A$-benzodiazepine receptor agonists**: zaleplon (Sonata), zolpidem (Ambien)
- **Barbiturates:** amobarbital (Amytal; *blues*), butabarbital (Butisol), butalbital (Fiorinal), pentobarbital (Nembutal; *yellow jackets*), phenobarbital (Luminal), secobarbital (Seconal; *reds*)
- **Older sedative-hypnotics** (much higher abuse potential; some discontinued, e.g., Quaalude): chloral hydrate, ethchlorvynol (Placidyl), ethinamate (Valmid), glutethimide (Doriden; *blues*), meprobamate (Equanil, Miltown), methyprylon (Noludar)

All the sedative-hypnotic drugs above are abusable and can produce dependency, even the safest of the classes such as long half-life benzodiazepines and zolpidem. Among this group of drugs, the benzodiazepines (and zolpidem) dominate clinical use. Most of the older drugs are highly addictive but fortunately are becoming increasingly uncommon. Any "minimum addictive dose" should be considered very approximate; there are marked individual differences. Recognize that some patients can become dependent on benzodiazepines when the drugs are used *in therapeutic doses*. The signs are often very subtle but very real. The risk for addiction increases with factors such as short-acting drugs; rapid onset of action; high doses; increased chronicity of use [1–2 months is usually safe but not always (particularly high-potency drugs), whereas 8–12 months poses a great risk for withdrawal even using benzodiazepines (perhaps 90% or more at therapeutic doses) (6)]; long-term "PRN" use [rather than continuous use—curious (7)]; nonbenzodiazepine drugs; concurrent alcoholism and polydrug abuse; chronic anxiety or dysphoria; and severe withdrawal effects (i.e., discomfort *and* a belief that the drug is required to treat the underlying condition).

Clinical Syndromes

The same variety of syndromes occurs with sedative-hypnotic abuse as occurs with alcohol. There is cross-tolerance between alcohol and the sedative-hypnotics and among the various drugs themselves. The clinical picture varies little from drug to drug (although withdrawal phenomena are more severe, but often briefer, with the shorter acting drugs).

SEDATIVE, HYPNOTIC, OR ANXIOLYTIC INTOXICATION (DSM-IV p. 263, 292.89)

Symptoms of intoxication are dose related. Mild intoxication includes a sense of well-being, talkativeness, irritability, and emotional disinhibition (uncommon; unpredictable). Increased doses produce apathy, confusion, stupor, and coma. Physical signs of intoxication include slurred speech, ataxic gait, incoordination, reduced DTRs, lateral nystagmus, and constricted pupils. Look for fast activity on the EEG. Fatalities are frequent with nonbenzodiazepine sedative-hypnotic ODs, usually due to respiratory depression. Benzodiazepine ODs generally are safe unless combined with another drug such as alcohol or an opiate.

Always evaluate sedative-hypnotic abusing patients who present with intoxication for an overt or covert OD. If they are becoming increasingly lethargic, treat as a medical emergency with hospitalization and intensive medical care. Obtain blood and urine levels.

SEDATIVE, HYPNOTIC, OR ANXIOLYTIC ABUSE (DSM-IV p. 263, 305.40)

This condition results from the pathologic use of one or more of this class of drugs for more than 1 month. These patients frequently cannot abstain from use, once started—a psychological addiction. Abuse of sedative-hypnotics is common. General cognitive impairment, anterograde amnesia, subtle psychomotor failings of which the patient is unaware, and mild to moderate depression become increasingly common the longer the drug is used, even at subintoxication doses. At least two distinct populations and patterns of abuse are recognized:

1. Males and females in their teens or 20s who obtain these drugs illegally and use them (as well as many other kinds) "for

fun" and to get high or to block things out and "get away from the hassle."

2. Middle-aged females (and males) who are frequently chronically anxious or depressed and who obtain legal prescriptions from (one or more) physicians for complaints of anxiety and insomnia, gradually increase the dosage themselves in an effort to cope, and often become physiologically addicted. Although these patients are common, they are seen most commonly by general physicians because they ultimately have to "doctor shop" to obtain drugs. Recognize them. Recognize also that these patients frequently vigorously deny their illness—both to their physicians *and*, sometimes, to themselves.

Without exception, if the patient takes enough drug long enough, he or she will develop tolerance to it and/or signs of physiologic withdrawal when it is stopped. If the patient *also* displays drug-seeking behavior and alters normal life activities to take the drug, then he or she has **SEDATIVE, HYPNOTIC, OR ANXIOLYTIC DEPENDENCE** (DSM-IV p. 262, 304.10). Most people are not "reinforced" by benzodiazepines and thus do not become dependent; alcoholics are the major exception. Some evidence suggests a familial pattern to the abuse of these substances (e.g., family members also abuse sedative-hypnotics and alcohol). Once detoxified, the sedative-hypnotic addict is more likely to "stay clean" if treated with an antidepressant or an anticonvulsant (such as carbamazepine, but not phenobarbital).

SEDATIVE, HYPNOTIC, OR ANXIOLYTIC WITHDRAWAL (DSM-IV p. 264, 292.0)

This may be the most dangerous of the drug withdrawal syndromes and can occur both in the dependent person who abstains and also in the person who merely reduces the dose. Its severity depends on the particular drug abused, the duration of use, the speed of discontinuation, and the daily dose used (degree of tolerance). Keep a high index of suspicion. It is often difficult to differentiate withdrawal from a marked worsening of symptoms due to *rebound anxiety*. Drugs such as alprazolam (used in high doses for panic disorder), lorazepam, and triazolam are particular offenders. Recognize withdrawal by (a) a history of significant drug use (*often* denied by the patient), (b) by characteristic abstinence symptoms (see below), and (c) by a tolerance test. The patients are typically very uncomfortable.

Withdrawal Symptoms

Psychological symptoms: a subjective sense of severe anxiety, restlessness, apprehension, irritability, insomnia, and anorexia that
has developed gradually over the past 24 hours (1–7 days with
the longer acting sedative-hypnotics) and is worsening hour by
hour. Delirium may occur (**SEDATIVE, HYPNOTIC, OR ANX-
IOLYTIC WITHDRAWAL DELIRIUM,** DSM-IV p. 131, 292.81)
with visual hallucinations and formication (sense of insects
crawling on the skin).

Physical symptoms: tremulousness (coarse tremor, primarily the
upper extremities), weakness, nausea and vomiting, orthostatic
hypotension, tachycardia, hyperreflexia, and diaphoresis. After several days this may progress to delirium, hyperpyrexia, and coma.
Seizures may occur (typically after 2–5 days), usually generalized
and single or a short series, but occasionally status epilepticus.

Tolerance Test   There are several methods of determining the
degree of dependence (and thus the probable severity and length
of withdrawal). One method is given below. It can be used regardless of the particular sedative-hypnotic drug of abuse (i.e., they are
all cross-tolerant).

1. Hospitalize the patient for the test if possible.
2. Administer the test to a patient who is comfortable or only
   mildly anxious (*not* to a patient who is intoxicated or
   presently withdrawing; the test would be invalid).
3. Give 200 mg of pentobarbital orally.
4. At 1 hour, evaluate the patient. If he or she is
   a. asleep but can be aroused, the patient has no tolerance.
   b. grossly ataxic, has a coarse tremor and nystagmus, daily
      tolerance is 400–500 mg of pentobarbital.
   c. mildly ataxic, mild nystagmus, daily tolerance is 600 mg.
   d. comfortable, with slight lateral nystagmus, daily toler-
      ance is 800 mg.
   e. asymptomatic or has continuing signs of mild with-
      drawal, daily tolerance is 1,000 mg *or more.* Wait 3–
      4 hours, then give an oral dose of 300 mg of pentobar-
      bital. Failure to become symptomatic at this larger dose
      suggests a daily tolerance of greater than 1,600 mg.

   Treat withdrawal vigorously and carefully. Usually hospitalize unless the addiction is mild and the patient reliable. Evalu-

ate for medical illness. Withdrawal can be accomplished safely using several different sedative-hypnotics (reliable iatrogenically addicted patients often are withdrawn with decreasing doses of their drug of abuse), although the most commonly used are diazepam, chlordiazepoxide, clonazepam, pentobarbital, and phenobarbital.

To withdraw with pentobarbital, give the estimated daily tolerance dose (obtained either by reliable history of all cross-tolerant drugs and alcohol used or by a tolerance test) equally divided on a q6 hour schedule for the first and second days and then reduce 10% of the initial dose each day. Expect the patient to be somewhat uncomfortable, but if signs of serious withdrawal (or intoxication) appear, slow (or quicken) the decrease slightly. Also expect a waxing and waning course as the detoxification proceeds. If the patient is showing serious withdrawal symptoms before treatment, give enough pentobarbital over several hours to make him or her comfortable and then begin the withdrawal procedure. The duration of the withdrawal may be as brief as 5–7 days for short-acting drugs and as long as a month or more for long-acting benzodiazepines.

SEDATIVE, HYPNOTIC, OR ANXIOLYTIC-INDUCED PERSISTING AMNESTIC DISORDER (DSM-IV p. 162, 292.83)

This profound, short-term, anterograde, and retrograde memory loss (Korsakoff's syndrome) is usually reversible.

HALLUCINOGENS

Drugs involved include (8)
1. **LSD-like**
   - lysergic acid diethylamide (LSD-25, *acid*)
   - dimethyltryptamine (DMT)
   - dimethoxymethylamphetamine (DOM, *peace, STP*)
   - 5-methoxy-3, 4-methylenedioxyamphetamine (MDMA, *ecstasy, XTC, X, Adam*) (9)
   - 3,4-methylenedioxyamphetamine (MDA)
   - Psilocybin
   - Mescaline (*peyote, tops, cactus*)
2. **Others**
   - phencyclidine (PCP, *angel dust, crystal, hog*)
   - thiocyclidine (TCP)

- ketamine (Ketalar)
- cannabis (marijuana, *hashish, pot, weed, grass, reefer*)
  delta-9-tetrahydrocannabinol (THC)

LSD, Mescaline, and Others

Patients take these drugs orally, develop symptoms in 10–45 minutes, and are back to normal in several hours (e.g., LSD) to 1–2 days. New synthetic drugs, with different characteristics, are created and "hit the streets" regularly, in both this class and among the stimulants: the world of *designer drugs.* The typical consequences of ingestion (**HALLUCINOGEN INTOXICATION,** DSM-IV p. 232, 292.89) are as follows.

Psychological symptoms: marked perceptual distortions (changing object shapes, changing body image), illusions and hallucinations (mostly visual geometric designs but also auditory and tactile), depersonalization, derealization, and synesthesias (stimuli in one modality produce sensations in another, e.g., sounds become colors)—all occurring in a clear sensorium. The patient is usually aware that what he is experiencing is due to drugs (i.e., has insight, unlike the patient with amphetamine psychosis). Occasionally the patient experiences strong depressive or anxious feelings (e.g., panic, "a bad trip"), but more typically the mood is euphoric and the patient feels he or she is receiving profound staggering insights [a "claim to fame" of ecstasy (10)].

Physical symptoms: tachycardia, palpitations, diaphoresis, pupillary dilation (responsive to light), blurred vision, tremor, incoordination, hyperreflexia, hyperthermia, and piloerection.

The psychological symptoms are particularly sensitive to the "set" or expectations of the patient before drug usage. Occasionally, the patient will experience brief hallucinations weeks, months, or even years after the period of drug use (**HALLU-CINOGEN PERSISTING PERCEPTION DISORDER,** DSM-IV p. 234, 292.89—*flashbacks*). Flashback frequency generally decreases with time but may continue for years, even in the absence of additional hallucinogen usage, *if* marijuana is used regularly. Although primarily recreational drugs, a few patients disrupt their lives with drug use (**HALLUCINOGEN ABUSE,** DSM-

IV p. 231, 305.30). There are no withdrawal symptoms, although slight tolerance does develop.

Two clinical syndromes that may (infrequently) follow the use of these drugs by one or more days are **HALLUCINOGEN-INDUCED PSYCHOTIC DISORDER, WITH DELUSIONS** (DSM-IV p. 314, 292.11), which are delusions that occur with drug use that may persist for a variable length of time after the drug is out of the body, and **HALLUCINOGEN-INDUCED MOOD DISORDER** (DSM-IV p. 375, 292.84), which is the persistence of depression or anxiety for days, weeks, or longer after taking the drug. The presentation may be identical to or gradually develop into a major mood disorder.

Treatment for "bad trips" usually consists of support ("talking down")—the patient usually clears within hours. Benzodiazepines and phenothiazines may be used briefly (e.g., diazepam 10–15 mg; haloperidol 4–5 mg) if patient is "wild."

Phencyclidine

PCP abuse (**PHENCYCLIDINE ABUSE,** DSM-IV p. 257, 305.90; **PCP DEPENDENCE,** 304.90) is most common among youth. PCP typically is eaten, taken IV, or (more recently) smoked. Symptoms begin in several minutes (smoked) or an hour or more (orally) and are dose dependent.

Psychological symptoms: low doses produce euphoria, grandiosity, a feeling of "numbness" and emotional lability. Higher doses cause symptoms that range from perceptual distortions, anxiety, excitation, confusion, and synesthesias to a paranoid psychosis, rigidity, and a catatonic-like state to convulsions, coma, and death. Violent (and self-destructive) behavior is probably rare (despite the reputation) either when intoxicated or perhaps several hours later during withdrawal.

Physical symptoms: tachycardia, hypertension, vertical and horizontal nystagmus, ataxia, dysarthria, myoclonus, decreased pain sensitivity, diaphoresis, and seizures.

The patient usually clears in 3–6 hours, but waxing and waning symptoms may last for days or longer with high doses. The symptom picture can be quite variable and can include a delirium lasting days but which may last weeks (**PHENCYCLIDINE INTOXICATION DELIRIUM,** DSM-IV p. 131, 292.81), delusions (**PCP-INDUCED PSYCHOTIC DISORDER, WITH DELUSIONS,** 292.11), or a varying organic mood disorder (**PCP-INDUCED MOOD DISORDER,** 292. 84). Long-term organic symptoms may occur (memory loss, word-finding difficulty), perhaps due to massive fat storage. Diagnosis is based on the clinical picture, a history of PCP use, the presence of PCP in urine, and (possibly) hair analysis (11). Chronic, denied PCP use can easily be misdiagnosed as "atypical psychosis," so be wary. Infants from addicted mothers often show hyperirritability, hypertonia, and delayed development that may last for months or even years.

Treatment is controversial. ODs can be fatal. Hospitalize and use gastric suction, urine acidification (ascorbic acid), fluids and diuretics, and symptomatic medical maintenance. If agitation must be controlled, consider diazepam or haloperidol. Decrease external stimulation.

Cannabis

The active ingredient of cannabis is THC. The various forms (e.g., marijuana, hashish) are all either smoked or eaten, and the differences in the effects they produce depend primarily on their concentrations of THC. Cannabis is used widely (daily alcohol and marijuana use are about equal among high school seniors; in a recent study, 20% of eighth-grade students have used marijuana), and a single dose usually produces mild physical and psychological alterations (**CANNABIS INTOXICATION,** DSM-IV p. 218, 292.89) that occur shortly after intake and last 2–4 hours.

Psychological symptoms: a sense of well-being, mild euphoria, and relaxation. Mild alterations and intensifications of perceptions occur (greater with the more concentrated forms), as does a sense of indifference and slowed time. A few persons find the use of cannabis dysphoric and develop depression, anxiety, panic, dissociation, or even a delusional syndrome (usually paranoid, often with depersonalization) (**CANNABIS-INDUCED PSYCHOTIC DISORDER, WITH DELUSIONS,** DSM-IV p. 314, 292.11). Impaired psychomotor performance, attention, time sense, and memory (ability to learn) during and shortly after use is common (expected); driving is dangerous. Chronic frequent use produces broad cognitive, and resulting social/occupational, impairment (12).

Physical symptoms: tachycardia, hypertension, *conjunctival injection,* dry mouth, and hunger. Chronic heavy use is carcinogenic.

Toxic psychoses have been reported with high-dose use. Some persons are socially and occupationally handicapped by chronic drug use (look for morning hangover) (**CANNABIS ABUSE,** DSM-IV p. 217, 305. 20). These patients are frequently apathetic and "amotivational," but this may be more a reflection of their personality structure than an effect of cannabis. If there is also a significant degree of tolerance (often develops quickly with heavy use) coupled with continued use despite impaired life functioning, the patient has **CANNABIS DEPENDENCE** (DSM-IV p. 216, 304.30). Dependence is more common than previously believed and occurs in about 10% of users (13). Withdrawal symptoms tend to be mild: irritability, anxiety, "flu-like."

Treat "bad trips" with support. Surreptitious use of marijuana can be detected up to several weeks after use by a urine screen for delta-9-THC-11-oic acid (THCA).

STIMULANTS

Drugs involved include
- amphetamine (Adderall, Benzedrine)
- dextroamphetamine (Dexedrine)
- methamphetamine [Desoxyn, Methedrine; snorted or swallowed (*speed, crystal*), smoked (*ice, glass*), IV (*crank*)]
- methylphenidate (Ritalin)
- phenmetrazine (Preludin)
- cocaine (including "crack")

These are effective orally (except cocaine) and nasally (cocaine) but produce a more rapid and intense effect by smoking [cocaine ("crack"), crystal methamphetamine ("ice")] and IV (an orgasm-like "rush"). Street terms for amphetamines include speed, bennies, uppers, diet pills, crystal, double crosses, crosstops, and ice; for cocaine include coke, snow, and crack (rock); and "speedball" for amphetamine or cocaine with an opioid. *Crack,* the alkaloidal free-base form of cocaine HCl, is inexpensive, widely available, and extremely addicting. Use of a new smokable form of methamphetamine (ice), which produces a cracklike effect, is spreading (14).

Clinical Syndromes

The effects of **AMPHETAMINE INTOXICATION** (DSM-IV p. 207, 292.89) and **COCAINE INTOXICATION** (DSM-IV p. 224, 292.89) occur within minutes (depending on route).

Psychological symptoms: of hyperalertness, restlessness, psychomotor agitation, pacing, talkativeness and pressure of speech, sense of well-being, and elation. Frequently aggressiveness, violent behavior, and poor judgment occur as well.

Physical symptoms: tachycardia, hypertension, pupillary dilation, chills and diaphoresis, anorexia, nausea and vomiting, and insomnia. Occasionally there are stereotyped repetitive movements (e.g., endlessly taking something apart and then reassembling it).

With brief use, symptoms usually disappear within hours of stopping the drug. All these symptoms may disappear as tolerance develops.

If drug use becomes a consuming pattern that lasts for at least 1 month and interferes with social and occupational functioning, the patient has **AMPHETAMINE ABUSE** (DSM-IV p. 206, 305.70) or **COCAINE ABUSE** (DSM-IV p. 223, 305.60). Abuse usually develops over months and may include a pattern of "runs" of frequent large-dose IV administration (amphetamines or crank) or smoking (crack) over days or weeks. After a run, the person frequently sleeps for 12–18 hours, then may begin another run. High-dose use places the patient at risk for developing:

- **AMPHETAMINE DEPENDENCE** (DSM-IV p. 206, 304.40): Tolerance and/or withdrawal coupled with major life changes.
- **AMPHETAMINE INTOXICATION DELIRIUM** (DSM-IV p. 131, 292.81): A characteristic organic delirium (see Chapter 5) develops shortly after taking the drug and disappears as the blood level drops. Violence is common during these episodes.
- **AMPHETAMINE-INDUCED PSYCHOTIC DISORDER, WITH DELUSIONS** (DSM-IV p. 314, 292.11): Patient becomes markedly paranoid and develops persecutory delusions within a setting of clear consciousness, often accompanied by hostility, anxiety, ideas of reference, and psychomotor agitation. This condition may last for 1 week or longer than 1 year. It easily

can be mistaken for paranoid schizophrenia, which it *closely* resembles.

- **AMPHETAMINE WITHDRAWAL** (DSM-IV p. 208, 292.0): Cessation of drug in the heavy user may be followed by mild-to-severe depression (watch for suicide), profound fatigue, irritability, anxiety, fearfulness, nightmares, and insomnia or hypersomnia. Severe symptoms seldom last more than 1 week but may be followed by chronic low-level depression and/or anxiety. Abnormal EEG patterns may last for weeks.

Cocaine produces similar syndromes. Serious medical complications occur with cocaine (particularly crack) and several can be fatal: MI (2° degree to coronary artery constriction; an MI in a young person is "due to cocaine until proven otherwise"), *crack lung* (acute "pneumonia" with normal x-ray and no response to routine medication), and anoxia 2° to seizures. Depression, paranoia and paranoid psychosis, marked anxiety, malnutrition, and pneumonia may follow use. Crack, when smoked, typically produces a high within seconds, followed by a dysphoric crash several minutes later, leading to rapidly repeated administrations and addiction. Infants of crack mothers are *jittery babies* who take weeks to gain weight, develop an appetite, and settle down but who then develop fairly normally except that many seem to become "hyperactive kids." It is a very bad drug. "Ice" is smoked similarly but produces a high lasting for hours—well on its way to becoming the new crack!

Make the diagnosis by the clinical picture and history of drug use. Most sympathomimetics and cocaine can be identified by a urine drug screen (cocaine is difficult—check with your laboratory).

Treatment

Stop the drug. If the patient is mildly or moderately excited, try to "talk him down" and use benzodiazepines (e.g., diazepam 10–20 mg PO). The patient may be agitated and violent, so take appropriate precautions (e.g., restraints). Treat severe intoxication, delirium, and delusional symptoms with an antipsychotic (e.g., haloperidol 10 mg PO or 5–10 mg IM). Acidify the urine with ascorbic acid or ammonium chloride (maintain pH at 4–5). Be alert to potential suicide and to medical complications (e.g., MI, stroke, intracranial hemorrhage). Severe withdrawal depressions may respond to antidepressants.

Cure is difficult. Consider hospitalization if symptoms or habit are severe or if life is severely disrupted. Group therapy (inpatient or outpatient) should be tried at some point. Desipramine (200–250 mg/day), bupropion, or amantadine (Symmetrel, 200–300 mg/day) may (?) decrease cocaine withdrawal cravings in a few, particularly depressed patients, yet neither medication nor formal psychotherapy has demonstrated prolonged effectiveness. There has been a moderately successful effort to use methylphenidate as a replacement medication (15).

INHALANTS

The types of glues, solvents, and cleaners "sniffed" for their psychic effects are numerous and include gasoline, kerosene, plastic and rubber cements, airplane and household glues, paints, lacquers, enamels, paint thinners, solvents, aerosols, furniture polishes, fingernail polish removers, nitrous oxide, and cleaning fluids, etc. Several active constituents are probably involved in most substances. This is a major abuse problem, particularly among young adolescents (begins at age 8–9, peaks at 14–15, disappears in most by age 20) and particularly among lower socioeconomic groups. It is often a group activity. Youth typically "grow out of it" (often moving to other drugs); addiction is very uncommon.

The effects from this variety of substance are usually quite similar, typically mild euphoria, giddiness, dizziness, slurred speech, confusion, disorientation, impulsivity, and ataxia—all of which may progress in the unusual case to a toxic psychosis, seizures, and coma (**INHALANT INTOXICATION,** DSM-IV p. 239, 292.89). Repeated and chronic abuse is common (**INHALANT ABUSE,** DSM-IV p. 238, 305.90), but withdrawal symptoms have not been noticed. Death has occurred from asphyxiation (e.g., confused child cannot remove a bag from his head), aspiration (usually vomit), dangerous behavior while intoxicated, and perhaps most commonly *sudden sniffing death syndrome* (child stimulated when high causes an outpouring of epinephrine that produces ventricular fibrillation in the inhalant-sensitized myocardium). An acute brain syndrome (delirium) often occurs, but only in the unusual or very severe case does the patient appear to develop a degree of chronic CNS damage. Toluene produces the greatest physical damage, including general CNS damage, hearing loss, and renal tubular necrosis. Chronic abuse, particularly of toluene, can result in CNS atrophy.

Physical restraint and medical support may be needed in the acute situation, but the patient usually clears over hours or days.

The nonintoxicated abuser often smells of solvent. Evaluate carefully for liver, kidney, and pulmonary damage. Encourage these children and their families to enter therapy.

NICOTINE

Nicotine in any form is highly addictive, producing both dependence (**NICOTINE DEPENDENCE,** DSM-IV p. 243, 305.10) and withdrawal (**NICOTINE WITHDRAWAL,** DSM-IV p. 244, 292.0—characterized by impaired concentration, irritability, restlessness, insomnia, hunger, and altered mood). On abrupt discontinuation, craving will begin within hours and then will continue for years (lifetime?). Abusers of multiple drugs typically report that nicotine is the most difficult drug to stop using permanently.

Treatment should be aimed at withdrawal and discontinuation, if the patient will allow it. When best done, this is a three-part process: (a) a behavioral smoking cessation program, (b) nicotine replacement and gradual dose decrease to keep craving tolerable, and (c) use of a drug specifically designed to decrease craving. A smoking cessation program (individual or group) seems to be essential for most patients. Nicotine replacement and titration is most commonly accomplished by nicotine gum (Nicorette; may need 25 or more pieces a day to start), a transdermal skin patch (Habitrol, Nicoderm, Nicotrol, ProStep), or a carefully monitored combination of the two. Finally, anticraving drugs remain of questionable value, with the best evidence suggesting mild usefulness for sustained release bupropion (Zyban) or clonidine (0.1–0.2 mg bid-tid). In addition, early evidence suggests that naltrexone, 50 mg/day, may reduce craving (16).

ANABOLIC STEROIDS

Not a problem in the "normal" doses used by patients with conditions like hypogonadism, anabolic steroids (most commonly testosterone and nandrolone) used in massive doses by athletes produce euphoria, irritability, and aggressiveness on use and depression on withdrawal. Approximately 25% of persons using supraphysiologic doses develop a major mood disorder at some point; a few become dangerously aggressive. There may be an association between steroid abuse and either antisocial or narcissistic personality disorder in some individuals (a worrisome combination regarding aggression) (17).

REFERENCES

1. Graham AW, Schultz TK, eds. *Principles of addiction medicine.* Chevy Chase, MD: American Society Addiction Medicine, 1998.
2. Ling W, Charuvastra VC, Kaim SC, et al. Methadyl acetate and methadone as maintenance treatments for heroin addicts. *Arch Gen Psychiatry* 1976;3:709–720.
3. Reynaud M, Petit G, Potard D, et al. Six deaths linked to concomitant use of buprenorphine and benzodiazepines. *Addiction* 1998;93: 1385–1392.
4. Schottenfeld RS, Pakes J, Ziedonis D, et al. Buprenorphine: dose-related effects on cocaine-abusing opioid dependent humans. *Biol Psychiatry* 1993;34:66–74.
5. Washton AM, Resnick RB. Clonidine for opiate detoxification: out-patient clinical trials. *Am J Psychiatry* 1980;137:1121–1122.
6. Rickels K, Schweizer E, Case G, et al. Long-term therapeutic use of benzodiazepines. I. Effects of abrupt discontinuation. *Arch Gen Psychiatry* 1990;47:899–907.
7. Roy-Byrne PP. Benzodiazepines: dependence and withdrawal. In: Roy-Byrne PP, Cowley DS, eds. *Benzodiazepines in clinical practice: risks and benefits.* Washington, DC: American Psychiatric Press, 1991;133– 153.
8. Abraham HD, Aldridge AM, Gogia P. The psychopharmacology of hallucinogens. *Neuropsychopharmacology* 1996;14:285–298.
9. Liester MB, Grob CS, Bravo GL, et al. Phenomenology and sequelae of 3,4-methylenedioxymethamphetamine use. *J Nerv Ment Dis* 1992; 180:345–352.
10. Cohen RS. Subjective reports on the effects of the MDMA ("ecstasy") experience in humans. *Prog Neuropsychopharmacol Biol Psychiatry* 1995;19:1137–1145.
11. Sramek JJ, Baumgartner WA, Tallos JA, et al. Hair analysis for detection of phencyclidine in newly admitted psychiatric patients. *Am J Psychiatry* 1985;142:950–953.
12. Pope HG, Todd-Yurgelun D. The residual cognitive effects of heavy marijuana use in college students. *JAMA* 1996;275:521–527.
13. Warner LA, Kessler RC, Hughes M, et al. Prevalence and correlates of drug use and dependence in the United States. *Arch Gen Psychiatry* 1995;52:219–229.
14. Baberg HT, Nelesen RA, Dimsdale JE. Amphetamine use: return of an old scourge in a consultation psychiatry setting. *Am J Psychiatry* 1996;153:789–793.
15. Grabowski J, Roache JD, Schmitz JM, et al. Replacement medication for cocaine dependence: methylphenidate. *J Clin Psychopharmacol* 1997;17:485–488.
16. Hutchison KE, Monti PM, Rohsenow DJ, et al. Effects of naltrexone with nicotine replacement on smoking cue reactivity. *Psychopharmacology* 1999;142:139–143.
17. Porcerelli JH, Sandler BA. Anabolic-androgenic steroid abuse and psychopathology. *Psychiatr Clin North Am* 1998;21:829–833.

Chapter 18

Psychosexual Disorders

These disorders are often first brought to the attention of the general physician. The three distinct categories are

- Psychosexual dysfunction—inhibition in sexual desire and/or psychophysiologic performance;
- Paraphilia—sexual arousal to deviant stimuli;
- Gender identity disorders—patient feels like the opposite sex.

PSYCHOSEXUAL DYSFUNCTION

Clinically observable features of the normal human *sexual response cycle* consist of four stages:

1. *Stage I: Excitement* (minutes to hours)
   - Males—psychological arousal and penile erection.
   - Females—psychological arousal, vaginal lubrication, nipple erection, and vasocongestion of the external genitalia.
2. *Stage II: Plateau* (seconds to 3 minutes)
   - Males—several drops of fluid appear at head of penis (from Cowper's gland).
   - Females—tightening of outer third of vagina, breast engorgement.
3. *Stage III: Orgasm* (5–15 seconds)
   - Males—ejaculation, involuntary muscular contraction (e.g., pelvis) followed by a refractory period.
   - Females—contractions of outer third of vagina, some involuntary pelvic thrusting; may be multiple.

4. *Stage IV: Resolution*
   - Males—relaxation, detumescence, sense of well-being.
   - Females—relaxation, detumescence, sense of well-being.

Patients (or their partners) may complain of decreased sexual desire and/or of one or more specific abnormalities of the response cycle. The dysfunctions may be situational, partial rather than complete, and primary or acquired. The phases usually occur in a stepwise fashion, but that is not mandatory—identify the stage involved. Often there are marital problems, unrealistic expectations, long-standing personal "hangups," chronic difficulty establishing and maintaining intimate interpersonal relations, etc. Identify these through history and psychiatric evaluation. *Always* evaluate carefully for organic causes (particularly with impotence and dyspareunia). Organic conditions tend to be chronic and independent of the situation.

Treatment should be global with an emphasis on intimacy and relationship, not just technique (1). Identify and treat psychosocial causes with dynamic psychotherapy, marital therapy, hypnotherapy, and group therapy. Sedatives may help temporarily if anxiety is prominent. Even purely physical causes often have significant associated secondary interpersonal problems that must be addressed once the medical condition has been corrected. A good prognosis is associated with acute recent dysfunction in a psychologically healthy patient with good past sexual functioning and strong sexual interests. Some relationships between partners are sufficiently hostile and destructive that unless other matters are resolved, prognosis is very poor for a correction of the psychosexual dysfunction.

The "new sex therapy" (Masters and Johnson) uses individual psychotherapy, couples therapy, education, behavior modification techniques, and often a male–female therapist pair (dual-sex therapy). Their numerous techniques have wide applicability with sexual dysfunctions and should be considered for use. Many of these methods center on decreasing a patient's (or couple's) anxiety about making love. Essential principles include

- Good communication with full exploration of sexual feelings;
- Training in specific stimulation and coital techniques (through "pleasuring sessions");
- Emphasis on the couple as a pleasure-giving team;

- Prohibition of intercourse early in therapy (to reduce performance anxiety);
- Emphasis on multimodal sensory pleasure (touch, sight, sound) and sensory awareness exercises;
- Insistence that physiologic responses be ignored (erection, etc.—"Don't worry about it; it will happen").

Male Erectile Disorder; Female Sexual Arousal Disorder (DSM-IV pp. 502 and 504, 302.72)

Males suffer *impotence:* a persistent or recurrent failure to reach or maintain a complete erection. Two forms exist: *primary impotence,* the patient has never maintained an erection, and *secondary impotence,* the patient has lost the ability—this may be person or situation specific (selective impotence).

Impotence is a common sexual complaint of men, predominantly the secondary form. It is *not* a "natural consequence" of aging. Some believe 90% of cases are psychogenic, but recent studies emphasize the frequency of an organic etiology. This is the most common sexual dysfunction caused by **SEXUAL DYSFUNCTION DUE TO A GENERAL MEDICAL CONDITION** (DSM-IV p. 518) or **SUBSTANCE-INDUCED SEXUAL DYSFUNCTION** (DSM-IV p. 521), although several other sexual problems can have an organic etiology as well. Organic causes include

- Disorders of the hypothalamic–pituitary–gonadal axis: Low serum testosterone level due to primary testicular hypofunction, pituitary tumors, etc.
- Endocrine: Hyperthyroidism (may have elevated testosterone), hyperprolactinemia, diabetes mellitus, acromegaly, Addison's disease, myxedema.
- Medication: TCAs, SSRIs (one-third or more of patients), MAOIs, major tranquilizers (particularly thioridazine), cholinergic blockers, antihypertensive drugs (particularly adrenergic blockers and false sympathetic neurotransmitters), estrogens, ethyl alcohol (alcoholism), addictive drugs (particularly narcotics and amphetamines), anticholinergic drugs.
- Illness: Any illness may cause impotence temporarily but particularly chronic debilitating disease, chronic renal disease,

peripheral vascular disease, and local physical and neurologic disorders (2).

Psychogenic causes include depression, anxiety (over cardiac status, performance, etc.), hostility and marital conflict, etc.

First identify any physical cause. Do a complete medical evaluation (look for physical illness, absent beard and body hair, small testes, gynecomastia) and get serum testosterone (then further hormonal studies if low). Early morning sleeping erection or occasional successful intercourse *does not rule out* an organic etiology, nor does a normal pattern of nocturnal penile tumescence (NPT—erections during REM sleep) *rule in* a psychogenic etiology, although most (all?) psychogenic cases have normal NPT. Treat medical causes (often curative). Follow with global therapy, if needed. Therapy includes allowing the female to play the dominant role and insisting on a gradual shift from foreplay to intercourse. Perhaps 30%–40% will not improve.

In **females**, an inadequate genital sexual response (failure to reach the excitement or plateau stages) is seen, although the woman *may* find sexual activity pleasurable. It often reflects personality or marital problems, but other specific causes include poor physical health, alcoholism, fatigue, depression, fear of pregnancy, and a postpartum state. Treat the couple. Pharmacologic understanding (e.g., testosterone replacement) is just beginning, but it *is* beginning (3).

PREMATURE EJACULATION (DSM-IV p. 511, 302.75)

The ejaculation occurs before the patient wishes it to and usually before his partner reaches orgasm (40% of all patients with sexual complaints; 30% of all males). Cause is often functional and secondary to anxiety (determine the source of the anxiety). It is much more common in stressful marriages. The "squeeze technique" can be effective: Just before ejaculation, the woman squeezes the head of glans. This is coupled with the man practicing imagery control. The young and vigorous male may benefit from 1% Nupercaine ointment applied to the coronal ridge and frenulum. Recently, selective serotonin reuptake inhibitors (SSRIs; e.g., fluoxetine 10 mg/day or more) have been found effective in many patients (4,5).

MALE ORGASMIC DISORDER (DSM-IV p. 509, 302.74)

The patient fails to ejaculate. Differentiate from *retrograde ejaculation* ("ejaculation" into the bladder—due to organic factors, e.g., anticholinergic drugs, prostatectomy). Some patients can have an orgasm only under certain conditions (e.g., with masturbation, with a stranger). Identify the circumstances in which orgasm can take place. Psychological causes include lack of interest (e.g., primary sexual deviation), anxiety, compulsive personality, marriage stresses, and sexual "hangups." Physical causes include medication [guanethidine, methyldopa, phenothiazines (particularly thioridazine), MAOIs, and one third or more of patients taking SSRIs], GU surgery, and lower spinal cord impairment (e.g., parkinsonism, syringomyelia). First train the patient to ejaculate by himself and then treat the interpersonal relationship—individual psychotherapy is often needed. The technique of the female self-inserting her partner's penis may be effective.

FEMALE ORGASMIC DISORDER (DSM-IV p. 506, 302.73)

The patient persistently fails to reach orgasm during intercourse. There are primary (the majority) and secondary forms, although be aware that many women become orgasmic as they get older (peak at age 35). There *may* be a biological basis in some (e.g., common with SSRIs), but most causes are psychological. This condition is very situation specific: Some women never have orgasm despite ample excitement, others have orgasm only with masturbation, still others require clitoral manipulation during intercourse, and some women can have an orgasm with intercourse alone. Psychotherapy often involves first training the woman to have an orgasm by herself and then treating the couple.

DYSPAREUNIA (DSM-IV p. 513, 302.76)

Pain with intercourse. It often is related to a physical condition (50%): cervical or vaginal infection or anatomic abnormality, endometriosis, tumor, or other pelvic pathology. Anxiety about sexual activity (for a variety of reasons) can produce pelvic muscle tightening and pain, but remember, pain from organic causes can produce anxiety, which exacerbates the pain. Also, dyspareunia can produce vaginismus, and vaginismus can produce dyspareunia.

VAGINISMUS (DSM-IV p. 515, 306.51)

During coitus, the patient has an involuntary spasm of the muscles surrounding the outer third of the vagina that prevents penile entrance. It may be related to physical causes producing pain—dyspareunia. Psychological causes include past sexual trauma (e.g., rape), a hostile marital relationship (perhaps from a vicious cycle), or sexual "hangups." Individual therapy and relaxation techniques are usually required. Hegar dilators (size increased over 3 to 5 days) may be useful.

HYPOACTIVE SEXUAL DESIRE DISORDER (DSM-IV p. 498, 302.71)

Common (20% of population, more female than male) and difficult to treat (6). It may present as inhibited excitement or inhibited orgasm—do not be misled. Causes often are functional. It varies with time, the sexual partner, depression, anxiety, and the stresses of the relationship. It may reflect a fear of intimacy or pregnancy, a passive-aggressive personality style, strong religious orthodoxy, or homosexuality, among others. Individual or couple therapy is useful. Testosterone replacement may be useful (e.g., methyltestosterone PO 0.25–1.0 mg/day) (7).

SEXUAL AVERSION DISORDER (DSM-IV p. 500, 302.79)

Similar to hypoactive sexual desire disorder but represents an *active* avoidance of sexual activity. Patient has often been sensitized by past (unpleasant) experiences.

PARAPHILIA (SEXUAL DEVIATION)

These patients become sexually excited only by unusual or bizarre stimuli (practices or fantasies) (8). The particular type of arousing stimulus determines the diagnosis. Orgastic release usually occurs by masturbation during or after the event. Etiology is uncertain but is possibly biologic, learned, and/or dynamic-instinctual. Most types are rare (courts see them most frequently), although physicians will occasionally encounter them. Men predominate, although women may display sadomasochism, voyeurism, and exhibitionism.

These patients may not be troubled by their desires (ego syntonic) and thus are difficult to treat, although depression, anxiety, and guilt do occur. These conditions frequently coexist with personality disorders, alcohol and drug abuse, and other psychiatric disorders—treat them. The patients often have impaired interpersonal relationships, particularly heterosexual relations.

Psychotherapy is frequently unsuccessful. Specific behavior modification and cognitive-behavioral techniques to eliminate the deviation may be useful (e.g., aversion – covert conditioning), although these must be paired with a more global retraining program (9). Hypersexual states and some other sexual deviations may benefit from medroxyprogesterone acetate (Depo-Provera) or cyproterone acetate (10), whereas some recent research suggests a possible use for fluoxetine and other antidepressants in decreasing aberrant drive (11,12).

PEDOPHILIA (DSM-IV p. 528, 302.2)

These patients repeatedly approach prepubertal children sexually (touch, explore, mutually masturbate; occasionally intercourse). They are usually anxious, depressed, inadequate males who know the child involved (a neighbor, relative). Three general types are recognized: *heterosexual pedophilia* (prefers preadolescent girls), *homosexual pedophilia* (prefers early teenage boys—very resistant to therapy), and mixed pedophilia (younger children, either sex). Pedophiliacs derive sexual arousal primarily from children: do not confuse with child molestation due to decreased impulse control (e.g., organic conditions, intoxication, retardation, psychosis) or a one-time event (e.g., due to loneliness or after a marital crisis). There may be biologic, familial roots. Behavior modification is the treatment of choice.

EXHIBITIONISM (DSM-IV p. 526, 302.4)

Usually timid males (onset usually in teen years) who become sexually aroused by exposing their genitals to an unsuspecting female (adult or child). They are only rarely aggressive. They may masturbate during the exposure and need a shock reaction from the female for satisfaction. Very resistant to treatment, although "compulsive" exhibitionism may respond to SSRIs.

Less frequent paraphilias include the following:

- **FETISHISM** (DSM-IV p. 526, 302.81): Sexual arousal to inanimate objects. May be combined with other sexual preferences.

- **FROTTEURISM** (DSM-IV p. 527, 302.89): Arousal from touching or fondling a nonconsenting person, usually in a crowded place where escape is possible. Usually teenage or young adult males.
- **TRANSVESTIC FETISHISM** (DSM-IV p. 531, 302.3): Aroused by female clothing and cross-dressing. Do not confuse with transsexualism (the wish to *become* a female) or effeminate homosexuality (cross-dressing to attract others, not to produce arousal itself).
- **VOYEURISM** (DSM-IV p. 532, 302.82): Sexual arousal by watching unsuspecting people who are naked or sexually active. Masturbation usually takes place concurrently.
- **SEXUAL MASOCHISM** (DSM-IV p. 529, 302.83): Arousal from being sexually bound, beaten, humiliated, etc. Chronic.
- **SEXUAL SADISM** (DSM-IV p. 530, 302.84): Sexual excitement after inflicting psychological or physical (sexual or nonsexual) harm on a consenting or nonconsenting partner. The severity of the harm required to produce excitement may increase with time, making the person a potential killer. Some rapists deserve this diagnosis.

GENDER IDENTITY DISORDER (DSM-IV p. 537)

These adults have experienced prolonged discomfort about their anatomic sex and identify with and wish they were the opposite sex. A few actively want to change their sex (transsexuals). Males predominate (M:F = 3:1), and their clinical characteristics are more variable. They may have experienced the discomfort since childhood or only recently. They may be homosexual, heterosexual, or have little sexual interest. Many have an effeminate appearance and cross-dress. Females with this disorder are usually homosexual and masculine appearing. Cross-dressing is common, there is *no* desire for a sex change, and there is a diversity of additional psychiatric symptomatology.

Etiology is unclear; it may be predominantly biologic and/or psychological, although the mother–child bond usually appears disturbed (often too close). Check karyotype and sex hormone levels. These patients are very likely to have personality disorders, particularly of the borderline type. The course is chronic, and there is significant risk for depression, suicide, anxiety, and genital self-mutilation. Rule out effeminate homosexuality (patient does *not* want to be the other sex), schizophrenia, and hermaphroditism.

Treat with supportive psychotherapy and feminizing-masculinizing hormones. Sex change surgery (castration, penectomy, vaginoplasty, phalloplasty) is falling out of fashion: It is irreversible and the results appear no better (perhaps worse) than psychotherapy alone (13,14). There have been isolated reports of gender identity changes with intensive behavior modification.

Homosexuality

Homosexuality [an arousal to and preference for sexual relations with adults of the same sex (15)] is not currently considered to be a mental disorder, except if the patient is "persistently and markedly" distressed by it (classed as **SEXUAL DISORDER NOT OTHERWISE SPECIFIED,** DSM-IV p. 538, 302.9). It may be a temporary phase during adolescence.

Homosexuality is common in the United States, with possibly 5%–10% of males and 2%–4% of females. Despite numerous theoretic explanations, the cause(s) is unknown. There may be congenital, prenatal, familial, biologic, and/or genetic [e.g., a gene on the X chromosome (16); debated by others (17)] etiologies for some; environmental factors may dominate in the choice of sexual orientation in others.

These distressed homosexuals often have internalized a negative attitude toward homosexual behavior and chronically and consistently want to change. They suffer from depression, anxiety, and shame. Psychotherapy for these symptoms may be helpful, but efforts at the patient's request to change sexual orientation has shown very limited long-term success.

REFERENCES

1. Cole M. Sex therapy—a critical appraisal. *Br J Psychiatry* 1985;147: 337–351.
2. Therapeutics and Technology Assessment Subcommittee. Assessment: neurological evaluation of male sexual dysfunction. *Neurology* 1995;45:2287–2292.
3. Bartlik B, Kaplan P, Kaminetsky J. Medications with the potential to enhance sexual responsivity in women. *Psychiatric Ann* 1999;29:46–52.
4. Haensel SM, Klem GMAL, Hop WCJ, et al. Fluoxetine and premature ejaculation. *J Clin Psychopharmacol* 1998;18:72–77.

5. Waldinger MD, Hengeveld MJW, Zwinderman AH, et al. Effect of SSRI antidepressants on ejaculation. *J Clin Psychopharmacol* 1998;18: 274–281.

6. Beck JG. Hypoactive sexual desire disorder: an overview. *J Consult Clin Psychol* 1995;63:919–927.

7. Bartlik B, Legere R, Andersson L. The combined use of sex therapy and testosterone replacement therapy for women. *Psychiatric Ann* 1999;29:27–33.

8. Abel GG, Osborn C. The paraphilias: the extent and nature of sexually deviant and criminal behavior. *Psychiatr Clin North Am* 1992;15: 675–687.

9. Hall GCN. Sexual offender recidivism revisited: a meta-analysis of recent treatment studies. *J Consult Clin Psychol* 1995;63:802–809.

10. Grossman LS, Martis B, Fichtner CG. Are sex offenders treatable? *Psychiatr Serv* 1999;50:349–361.

11. Stein DJ, Hollander E, Anthony DT, et al. Serotonergic medications for sexual obsessions, sexual addictions, and paraphilias. *J Clin Psychiatry* 1992;53:267.

12. Zohar J, Kaplan Z, Benjamin J. Compulsive exhibitionism successfully treated with fluvoxamine. *J Clin Psychiatry* 1994;55:86–88.

13. Snaith P, Tarsh MJ, Reid R. Sex reassignment surgery. *Br J Psychiatry* 1993;162:681–685.

14. Brown GR. A review of clinical approaches to gender dysphoria. *J Clin Psychiatry* 1990;51:57–64.

15. Cabaj RP, Stein TS. *Textbook of homosexuality and mental health.* Washington, DC: American Psychiatric Press, 1996.

16. Hamer DH, Hu S, Magnuson VS, et al. A linkage between DNA markers on the X chromosome and male sexual orientation. *Science* 1993;261:321–327.

17. Rice G, Anderson C, Risch N, et al. Male homosexuality: absence of linkage to microsatellite markers at Xq28. *Science* 1999;284:665–667.

Chapter 19

Sleep Disturbances

Sleep disorders are extremely common: 40% of the population have had trouble sleeping within the past year, 10% have had diagnosable insomnia, and 3%–4% have had hypersomnia (1–3).

Current understanding and classification of sleep problems rests on knowledge of normal sleep. Much of this has been obtained through *polysomnography* (4), that is, electrophysiologic measures [EEG, EMG, EOG], as well as airflow, O_2 saturation, etc., of patients in sleep laboratories. The two major categories are the **dyssomnias** (poor sleep, excessive sleep) and the **parasomnias** (peculiar events associated with sleep).

NORMAL SLEEP

Normal sleep is cyclical (4–5 cycles/night) and active, *not* passive. Distinct stages [rapid-eye-movement (REM) and non-REM sleep], measured by EEG, occur each night. From *waking* (beta waves; alpha waves, 8–12 cps), sleep is initiated by melatonin release from the pineal gland and passes stepwise through discrete stages during the night:

NREM Sleep: Low level of activity—lowered BP, heart rate, temperature, and respiratory rate. Good muscle tone and slow, drifting eye movements.

Stage 1—(*5%* of sleep), lightest sleep, a transition stage; low voltage, desynchronized waves.

Stage 2—(*50%*), mostly theta waves (low voltage, 5–7 cps) but with some bursts of *sleep spindles* (13–15 cps for 2–3 seconds) and high spikes (*K complexes*); awakens easily.

Stage 3—theta with some delta waves (high voltage at 0.5–2.5 cps).
Stage 4—deepest sleep (hard to awake), mostly in first half of
night; mostly delta waves.
REM Sleep: (*20%–25%* of sleep), active sleep characterized by
rapid synchronous eye movement, twitching of facial and extremity muscles, penile erections, and variation in pulse, BP, and
respiratory rate. Muscles appear *paralyzed* (no tone). Depth is
similar to stage 2; theta waves, sleep spindles, and K-complexes
reappear. *Dreaming* can occur in several stages but is most
common in REM sleep. Brain activity is quite elevated.

Patients enter lightest sleep (stage 1), descend by steps over
approximately 30 minutes to deepest sleep (stage 4), plateau there
for 30–40 minutes, and then ascend to lighter stages (1–2) to enter
REM sleep 90–100 minutes after falling asleep. Then the cycle
repeats. As the night progresses, the REM periods lengthen, stage
4 disappears, and the sleep is generally lighter. The length of time
spent in any one stage varies in a characteristic fashion with age
(e.g., longer stages 3 and 4 in youth, shorter and fewer in old age).
The significance of each stage is not known. Serum cortisol is low
initially during the night but peaks just before awakening.

For clinical purposes, patients can be divided into those complaining of insomnia or hypersomnia. In each category, there are
distinct syndromes that must be ruled in or out.

INSOMNIA

PRIMARY INSOMNIA (DSM-IV p. 557, 307.42)

Primary insomnia is persistent insomnia that has been present for
at least 1 month and has no obvious cause. Explore the differential diagnosis. Take a good history of the sleep problem; include
the 24-hour sleep–wake cycle (sleep laboratory studies usually are
not needed). Identify the pattern: trouble falling asleep (onset
insomnia), trouble staying asleep (frequent awakenings), early
morning awakenings (terminal insomnia). Inquire about life
stresses, drug and alcohol use, marital and family problems. Rule
out the following:

- Is the insomnia simply normal sleep?
  a. Some "insomniacs" get ample sleep (*sleep-state misperception syndrome* or *pseudoinsomnia*), they just believe they sleep poorly. Use reassurance and psychotherapy.
  b. Sleep time lessens with age—explain to concerned elderly. Help them avoid a "worry over sleeplessness" cycle.
  c. Some patients are substance abusers seeking drugs; do not be fooled.
- Is the insomnia transient (*situational insomnia*)? This is the most common form of insomnia: usually trouble falling asleep, due to worry. Identify the stress. Help the patient deal with it. Consider time-limited (1–2 weeks) use of sleeping medication (e.g., zolpidem, 5–10 mg PO, HS; temazepam, 15–30 mg PO, HS). Differentiate from *psychophysiological* or *conditioned insomnia:* The patient has inadvertently *trained* him or herself to stay awake at bedtime, usually by worrying about not falling asleep (a type of 1° insomnia).
- Is there a *chronic minor psychiatric illness?* Prolonged insomnia (usually sleep onset problems with decreased stage 4 sleep) is common with chronic depression and/or anxiety (and obsessive-compulsive patients). They may self-medicate, producing more insomnia. Such patients may have trouble expressing distressed or aggressive feelings and thus internalize their problems.
- Is there a major psychiatric illness (**INSOMNIA RELATED TO ANOTHER MENTAL DISORDER,** DSM-IV p. 596, 307.42)?
  a. *Acute psychosis:* Often produces major sleep disruption—use antipsychotics.
  b. *Mania or hypomania:* Very short sleep time—use anticonvulsants or lithium.
  c. *Major depression:* Typically early morning awakening, but frequent awakenings during the night are also common. REM sleep begins very quickly after sleep onset (*short REM latency*). Treat the depression with SSRIs, etc.
- Is there a medical problem (**SLEEP DISORDER DUE TO A GENERAL MEDICAL CONDITION, INSOMNIA TYPE,** DSM-IV p. 600, 780.52)?

a. Nighttime pain or distress, often with related anxiety and depression, e.g., back pain, headache, arthritis, asthma, nocturnal angina (increased chest pains during REM sleep), duodenal ulcer.

b. Hyperthyroidism, epilepsy, parkinsonism, chronic renal failure.

c. Is the patient simply worried about a medical problem?

- Is there substance use or abuse (**SUBSTANCE-INDUCED SLEEP DISORDER,** DSM-IV p. 606)? Very common so always inquire.

    a. Alcohol—The most common self-prescribed hypnotic. Intoxication yields heavy sleep for 2–4 hours; then restless dream-filled sleep. Chronic use produces increasingly fragmented sleep after initial sedation. Withdrawal generates intense REM sleep with vivid dreams.

    b. Hypnotic medication—Often prescribed for insomnia, it produces decreased REM sleep. Tolerance develops to each type with, ironically, sleep disruption ("sleeping-pill insomnia"). Severe rebound insomnia usually occurs with withdrawal. Treatment *must* begin with medication withdrawal—one therapeutic dose per week.

    c. Amphetamines, methylphenidate, cocaine, caffeine (patients often overlook; insomnia *particularly* in the elderly; ask), hallucinogens, aminophylline, ephedrine, thyroid, and steroids all can interrupt sleep. Usually hypersomnia with withdrawal.

    d. Cigarettes (nicotine) can stimulate; a commonly overlooked explanation.

- Is there *sleep cycle disruption* (**CIRCADIAN RHYTHM SLEEP DISORDER,** DSM-IV p. 578, 307.45)? Sleepiness slips out of phase if there is "jet lag" or night shift work; most commonly patients fall asleep (finally) in early morning and waken around noon or early afternoon. Usually self-limited, but improved sleep can be hastened by forced awakening and exposure to bright light increasingly earlier in the morning. Bright morning light on the retina sends a signal through the retinohypothalamic tract to the ventrolateral parts of the suprachiasmatic nuclei (SCN; the brain's circadian "pacemaker"; in the anterior hypothalamus). The impulse from this light causes the SCN to stimulate the pineal gland to *decrease* output of **melatonin,** causing alertness. With darkness, melatonin increases, causing sleepiness and feeding back to the SCN, which has melatonin receptors. Thus, bright light every morning uses this SCN–melatonin feedback loop to reset our brain's automatic internal clock located in the SCN. Melatonin *may* become a help with jet lag and other sleep rhythm disorders (5).

- Is there **DYSSOMNIA NOS** (DSM-IV p. 579, 307.47)? Could it be *periodic limb movement of sleep* (nocturnal myoclonus): restless sleep with frequent awakenings secondary to rhythmic (every 20–60 seconds) muscle jerks in the legs? Ask the bed partner. However, recent evidence suggests that nocturnal myoclonus rarely awakens the patient (only the partner). Onset around puberty; autosomal dominant. Best treatment at this point seems to be pergolide (6), although low-dose benzodiazepines may help. Or could insomnia be caused by the *restless legs syndrome?* Legs feel "uncomfortable," strong urge to move the legs; feeling relieved by moving. About 5% of population; more common in elderly. Treat with pramipexole (7) (1.5 mg 1–2 hours before bed), pergolide (8) (0.5 mg 1–2 hours before bed), or maybe carbidopa/levodopa (9).

- Are there *parasomnias,* e.g., frequent *nightmares* (**NIGHTMARE DISORDER,** DSM-IV p. 583, 307.47), *night terrors* (*pavor nocturnus;* **SLEEP TERROR DISORDER,** DSM-IV p. 587, 307.46), or *sleepwalking* (*somnambulism;* **SLEEPWALKING DISORDER,** DSM-IV p. 591, 307.46)?

  a. Nightmares (REM sleep) can be chronic and disruptive. They are common in children (25%–50%) but often disappear by adulthood; F:M = 2–4:1. Psychotherapy *may* help.

  b. Night terrors (stage 4 sleep) occur early in the night in children, are terrifying to observers, but are not remembered by the patient. They usually disappear with adulthood. Some respond to low doses of minor tranquilizers or SSRIs (10).

  c. Somnambulism (stage 4 sleep) can persist into adulthood. The patient's behavior appears strange to an observer; there is marked clouding of consciousness. Protect the patient from his or her actions. Diazepam 15 mg HS, imipramine 50 mg HS, or SSRIs may help.

General Treatment of Insomnia

1. Rule out, or treat, specific syndromes.
2. Practice good *sleep hygiene*. Maintain a regular bedtime; use bedroom for sleeping only. Keep room dark, quiet, and cool. Develop a "sleeping ritual" for the hour before going to bed. Arise about the same time every morning (*very* important). Regular exercise during the day helps, but not after dinner. Avoid vigorous mental activities late in the evening. Try a bedtime snack (yes, warm milk helps–tryptophan) but *do not* drink alcohol after supper or caffeine after mid-afternoon.** If not asleep after 30 minutes, get up and read or watch television until sleepy again, but still rise at the regular time in the morning, even if it produces daytime sleepiness for a few days (sleep restriction).**
3. Provide support and reassurance. Use psychotherapy, if there are issues. Try relaxation techniques: progressive relaxation, biofeedback, self-hypnosis, meditation, etc. Emphasize a sense of self-control.
4. Use sedative-hypnotics for a limited time only (see Chapter 23). Most hypnotic medications become ineffective within 2 weeks if used nightly. Try initially for 1 week in an effort to establish a successful sleep pattern (e.g., flurazepam 15–30 mg PO, HS but be aware that flurazepam can produce a gradual worsening of psychomotor performance during day). If used longer than a week, introduce drug holidays or use 2–3 times/week and do not exceed recommended dosages.

HYPERSOMNIA

PRIMARY HYPERSOMNIA (DSM-IV p. 562, 307.44)

Patients with *primary hypersomnia* sleep 10–12 hours at night and typically are sleepy and nap during the day. Their hypersomnia often starts in later teens; polygraph tracings are normal. They may make up 1%–2% of the population. Sleep often provides an escape from stress. Depression also occurs but is not typical, unlike its common presence in **HYPERSOMNIA RELATED TO**

ANOTHER MENTAL DISORDER, DSM-IV p. 597, 307.44. Key differential conditions include the following.

NARCOLEPSY (DSM-IV p. 567, 347)

Narcolepsy is a lifelong disorder (minimum requirement for diagnosis is 3 months) of brief, frequent, *refreshing* episodes of daytime sleep that usually begins near or shortly after puberty, has a genetic component [10% of 1° relatives; 90%–100% have a specific histocompatibility (HLA) antigen], occurs with a frequency of about 1 in 2,000 (0.05%), and requires (a) below as well as one or more of (b) through (d). About 15% of patients experience the whole *narcoleptic tetrad* (number of symptoms increase with middle age):

a. Daytime *sleep attacks*—The patient falls asleep in seconds or minutes (REM activity on EEG) during the day despite efforts to stay awake. The patient usually sleeps for 10–30 minutes and wakes refreshed, typically experiencing a single to a dozen episodes a day. Attacks occur most often during "slow times" but can happen while the patient is active and engaged (during a speech, driving a car) and can be embarrassing or dangerous.

b. *Cataplexy* (70% of patients)—A sudden loss of muscle tone, usually in the face and neck, but occasionally a complete physical collapse, typically precipitated by a strong emotion (e.g., anger, laughter). Attacks usually last for seconds and may be weeks apart. The patient is conscious throughout.

c. *Hypnagogic hallucinations* (30% of patients)—Dreamlike and often frightening auditory and/or visual hallucinations (REM on EEG) that occur as the patient falls asleep (or awakens—*hypnopompic*).

d. *Sleep paralysis* (25% of patients)—A flaccid, generalized, terrifying paralysis lasting for several seconds in a fully conscious patient, either while waking or falling asleep. It may resolve spontaneously or when the patient is touched or his or her name is called.

Many patients with narcolepsy also have disturbed nighttime sleep with frequent awakenings and nightmares. Diagnosis usually is not hard: Along with the classic tetrad, there is a remarkably short latency between falling asleep and REM sleep.

Treatment

- Train the patient to avoid dangerous occupations and precipitating stimuli. Planned daytime naps (15–30 minutes) can help.
- Sleep attacks—methylphenidate (Ritalin), 5–15 mg PO tid; dextroamphetamine (Dexedrine), 5–15 mg PO tid; a new medication modafinil (Provigil), 200 mg q A.M. Try occasional drug holidays. Medication advances are on the horizon (11).
- Cataplexy—imipramine, 10–25 mg PO tid, or fluoxetine, 20 mg/day (suppresses REM sleep).
- Consider sedation for nighttime insomnia (i.e., benzodiazepines); use sparingly.

Sleep Apnea (BREATHING-RELATED SLEEP DISORDER, DSM-IV p. 573, 780.59)

This set of serious nighttime respiratory abnormalities can cause long-standing daytime sleepiness, particularly during quiet times (not during stimulation, like narcolepsy). It occurs in three types:

1. A few patients, usually elderly, briefly cease nighttime breathing efforts due to abnormal chemoreceptors and develop repeated air hunger and *insomnia* (*Central Sleep Apnea*).
2. Most considered to have sleep apnea struggle to draw air through relaxed, flaccid nose and mouth passageways that have markedly increased sleep-induced resistance (*Obstructive Sleep Apnea*). There may be from 30 to several hundred episodes each night lasting from 10 seconds to more than 2 minutes. Males are affected 10:1 [look for obese men (majority of these patients) over age 50 with short thick necks]. The patients may experience a variety of symptoms, including *loud snoring, morning headaches, restless sleep,* frequent awakenings, impaired libido, sleepwalking, hypertension, depression, and intellectual and personality changes. Only a few cases will demonstrate fixed anatomic abnormalities of upper airway structures, but in many with weight gain and thickened necks, abnormalities appear during sleep. In serious chronic cases, pulmonary hypertension (12), right heart failure, and/or cardiac arrhythmias may occur. The polysomnograph shows fragmented sleep with frequent awakenings.

3. *Mixed Sleep Apnea*—suffering both phenomena.

No treatment has been clearly effective for central sleep apnea. A permanent tracheotomy or other surgical procedure (13) may be dramatically successful in obstructive sleep apnea, but try weight loss and/or continuous positive airway pressure (CPAP) first. Hypnotics can further compromise nighttime breathing, so avoid them. This important diagnosis is significantly underrecognized (14) and can mimic depression, anxiety, panic disorder, and early dementia.

Other Causes

Rule out current chronic overuse of sedative drugs and alcohol, or rebound in chronic stimulant users. Rule out medical conditions (**SLEEP DISORDER DUE TO A GENERAL MEDICAL CONDITION, HYPERSOMNIA TYPE,** DSM-IV p. 600, 780.54), e.g., myxedema, hypercapnia, any brain tumor but particularly those involving the mesencephalon and walls of the third ventricle, seizures, cerebrovascular disease, and hypoglycemia. Severe hypersomnia with marked postawakening confusion occurs with both the Pickwickian syndrome (obesity and respiratory insufficiency) and the Kleine-Levin syndrome (attacks of hyperphagia, hypersomnia, and hypersexuality).

REFERENCES

1. Chokroverty S. *Sleep disorders medicine: basic science, technical considerations, and clinical aspects.* Boston: Butterworth, 1999.
2. Kryger MH, Roth T, Dement WC. *Principles and practice of sleep medicine.* Philadelphia: W.B. Saunders, 1994.
3. Reite M, Ruddy J, Nagel K. *Evaluation and management of sleep disorders.* Washington, DC: American Psychiatric Press, 1997.
4. Reite M, Buysse D, Reynolds C, et al. The use of polysomnography in the evaluation of insomnia. *Sleep* 1995;18:58–70.
5. Silver R, LeSauter J, Tresco P, et al. A diffusible coupling signal from the transplanted suprachiasmatic nucleus controlling circadian locomotor rhythms. *Nature* 1996;382:810–814.
6. Silber MH. Restless legs syndrome. *Mayo Clin Proc* 1997;72:261–264.
7. Montplaisir J, Nicolas A, Denesle R, et al. Restless legs syndrome improved by pramipexole. *Neurology* 1999;52:938–943.
8. Wetter TC, Stiasny K, Winkelmann J, et al. A randomized controlled study of pergolide in patients with restless legs syndrome. *Neurology* 1999;52:944–950.

9. Earley CJ, Allen RP. Pergolide and carbidopa/levodopa treatment of the restless legs syndrome and periodic leg movements in sleep in a consecutive series of patients. *Sleep* 1996;19:801–810.

10. Lillywhite AR, Wilson SJ, Nutt DJ. Successful treatment of night terrors and somnambulism with paroxetine. *Br J Psychiatry* 1994;164: 551–554.

11. Mitler MM, Aldrich MS, Koob GF, et al. ASDA standards of practice: practice parameters for the use of stimulants in the treatment of narcolepsy. *Sleep* 1994;17:348–351.

12. Chaouat A, Weitzenblum E, Krieger J, et al. Pulmonary hemodynamics in the obstructive sleep apnea syndrome. *Chest* 1996;109:380–386.

13. ASDA Standards of Practice Committee. Practice parameters for the treatment of obstructive sleep apnea in adults: the efficacy of surgical modifications of the upper airway. *Sleep* 1996;19:152–155.

14. Reite M. Sleep disorders presenting as psychiatric disorders. *Psychiatr Clin North Am* 1998;21:591–607.

Chapter 20

Personality Disorders

Personality is a consistent style of behavior uniquely recognizable in each individual. *Personality disorders* (Axis II of DSM-IV p. 633) refers to personality characteristics of a form or magnitude that are unchanging, chronic, occur in most settings, deviate significantly from cultural norms, and are maladaptive and cause poor life functioning (1). Many patients display a mixture of several different maladaptive traits. These *long-term* traits feel "natural" (ego syntonic), even though a person may be bothered by the results of his or her behavior. There are elements of the personality disorders in all of us, and the difference between health and pathology may be one of degree. Moreover, many patients only display their pathology clearly when under stress.

Most personality disorders begin to take shape in childhood and become fixed by the early 20s, yet some occur after organic insults to the brain. Some may have a biologic, and even a genetic (2,3), component (e.g., schizotypal and borderline personality disorders). Psychological testing may facilitate diagnosis (i.e., WAIS, MMPI, Bender-Gestalt, and Rorschach). Atypical and mixed types are common, and some may grade into or be confused with similar appearing Axis I disorders (e.g., paranoid personality disorders look like paranoid schizophrenia). These patients often resist treatment and change slowly but occasionally respond to a variety of treatment modalities, including individual or group therapy and short-term use of antianxiety agents or low doses of major tranquilizers (4,5). Some may require inpatient treatment during periods of decompensation. Adolescents (under 18), and even children, may receive a personality disorder diagnosis (except antisocial personality disorder) if the pattern is stable, clear, and incompatible with an Axis I childhood disorder.

The ten personality disorders are divided into three distinct groups ("clusters") based on their clinical patterns: the *odd eccentric* cluster, the *dramatic, emotional, and erratic* cluster, and the *anxious, fearful* cluster. They are as their names suggest.

ODD ECCENTRIC CLUSTER

PARANOID PERSONALITY DISORDER (DSM-IV p. 634, 301.0)

These aloof emotionally cold people typically display unjustified suspiciousness, hostility, hypersensitivity to slights, jealousy, and a fear of intimacy. They tend to be grandiose, rigid, unforgiving, sarcastic, contentious, and litigious and are thus isolated and disliked. They accept criticism poorly, blaming others instead. This disorder may be associated with chronic CNS impairment, drug use (e.g., amphetamines), depression, obsessive-compulsive states, or as a precursor to schizophrenia. Psychotic decompensation sometimes occurs, requiring major tranquilizers. They rarely seek treatment, and therapy, including medication, is of little value.

SCHIZOID PERSONALITY DISORDER (DSM-IV p. 638, 301.20)

These are seclusive people who have little wish or capacity to form interpersonal relations, are indifferent to and derive little pleasure from social and sexual contacts, and yet prefer and can perform well at solitary activities (e.g., night watchman). They have a limited emotional range, experience little pleasure, daydream excessively, and are humorless and detached. They do *not* seem to have an increased risk of developing schizophrenia as was previously thought. "Loners" are not necessarily schizoid unless they have impaired functioning. Treatment seems of little help.

SCHIZOTYPAL PERSONALITY DISORDER (DSM-IV p. 641, 301.22)

In addition to having features of the schizoid (isolated, anhedonic, aloof), these people are "peculiar." They relate strange intrapsychic experiences, display odd and magical beliefs as well as strange speech, reason in odd ways (e.g., ideas of reference), are frequently anxious, and are difficult to "get to know," yet none of these features reach psychotic proportions. It is found in 3% of the population, commonly co-occurs with major depression, and is associated with an increased incidence of schizophrenia in family members (suggesting that this condition is part of the "schizophrenic spectrum" of disorders). Biologic measures found in schizophrenia also occur [e.g., impaired eye tracking (6) and increased CSF homovanillic acid (7)]. Low-dose antipsychotic medication may reduce the more flamboyant symptoms.

DRAMATIC, EMOTIONAL, AND ERRATIC CLUSTER

ANTISOCIAL PERSONALITY DISORDER (DSM-IV p. 645, 301.7)

Antisocial behavior begins in childhood or early adolescence: aggressiveness, fighting, "hyperactivity," poor peer relationships, irresponsibility, lying, theft, truancy, poor school performance, runaway, inappropriate sexual activity, and drug and alcohol use. As adults there is criminality, assaultiveness, self-defeating impulsivity, hedonism, promiscuity, unreliability, and crippling drug and alcohol abuse. They fail at work, change jobs frequently, go AWOL and receive dishonorable discharges from the service, are abusing parents and neglectful mates, cannot maintain intimate interpersonal relationships, and spend time in jails and prisons (50% or more of prisoners). These patients are frequently, if temporarily, anxious and depressed (suicide, often impulsive, in as many as 5%) and are second only to patients with hysteria in the production of conversions symptoms. The behavior peaks in late adolescence and the early 20s with improvement in the 30s; however, the patients usually continue their antisocial patterns and they rarely recover from the "lost years." Males are involved more severely, earlier, and more frequently (3% of population); M:F = 3–5 : 1.

Their rearing is generally impaired by rejection, neglect, desertion, poverty, and inconsistent discipline; they are frequently illegitimate and unwanted. The parents are often criminals (30% of fathers), alcoholics (50% of fathers), and chronically unemployed. Male first-degree relatives have an increased incidence of antisocial personality disorder, alcoholism, and drug abuse, and female relatives have associated somatization disorder. A genetic component is likely.

No tests are diagnostic, although a 4–9 MMPI profile is common, and there is an increased incidence of nonspecific EEG abnormalities (increased slow-wave activity, etc.). It is necessary to rule out primary drug and alcohol abuse (difficult, look for normal childhood behavior), schizophrenia (thought disorder present), OBS (disorientation, memory impairment), early mania, explosive disorder, and **ADULT ANTISOCIAL BEHAVIOR** (DSM-IV p. 683, V71.01). Several very specialized disorders of impulse control can also mimic this disorder: **PATHOLOGICAL GAMBLING** (DSM-IV p. 615, 312.31), **KLEPTOMANIA** (DSM-IV p. 612.32), and **PYROMANIA** (DSM-IV p. 614, 312.33). The patients are resistant and manipulative. Do not rely on the patient's report; check your data. They rarely seek help for personality change, and treatment is difficult and often unsuccessful. Best results follow closely supervised inpatient care: Use strong, frequent, and accurate confrontation of interpersonal behavior, particularly by peers. Individual outpatient psychotherapy is of little value. The terms antisocial personality disorder, sociopathy, and psychopathy generally [but not always (8)] are used synonymously.

BORDERLINE PERSONALITY DISORDER (DSM-IV p. 650, 301.83)

These usually socially adapted patients have complex clinical presentations, including diverse combinations of anger and sarcasm, anxiety, intense and labile affect, brief disturbances in consciousness (e.g., depersonalization, dissociation), chronic loneliness, boredom, a chronic sense of emptiness, unstable and volatile interpersonal relations, identity confusion, impulsive behavior (including self-injury–cutting and self-mutilation; recurrent suicide attempts; and death by suicide in 8% or more), and a *hypersensitivity to abandonment.* Stress can precipitate a transient psychosis. Many other diagnoses are often suggested or can also be made: depression, brief psychotic disorder, other personality disorders, cyclothymic disorder, and substance-related disorders. Some of this common (2% in general population; F:M = 3:1) heterogeneous group may be related genetically to affective disorders or schizophrenia and others to subtle organic deficits, whereas specific symptoms may be related to specific neurotransmitters (e.g., impulsivity and low CNS serotonin). There is often, but *not* always, a history of early childhood abuse. Psychological testing is useful. Be sure to rule out organic states such as mild delirium, psychomotor epilepsy, or drug use in the acute presentation. Long-term, intermittent, supportive psychotherapy is often beneficial, although *numerous* other psychotherapies have their supporters. Low-dose antipsychotic agents (thioridazine 100–300 mg HS, haloperidol 4–6 mg HS) for short periods, antidepressants (SSRIs, MAOIs), or lithium carbonate may help selected individuals. These patients tend to stabilize in their 40s and 50s.

HISTRIONIC PERSONALITY DISORDER (DSM-IV p. 655, 301.50)

Histrionic patients initially seem charming, likable, lively, and seductive but gradually become seen as emotionally unstable, egocentric, immature, dependent, manipulative, excitement-seeking, and shallow. They demand attention, are exhibitionistic and suggestible, and present a "caricature of femininity" yet have a limited ability to maintain stable, intimate, interpersonal relationships with either sex. This common disorder (2% or more in general population) is associated with depression, substance abuse, and conversion and (particularly) somatization disorders. Suicidal gestures and attempts are common. Lesser impaired patients respond to psychotherapy.

NARCISSISTIC PERSONALITY DISORDER (DSM-IV p. 658, 301.81)

Although often symptom free and well functioning, these patients are chronically dissatisfied due to a constant need for admiration and habitually unrealistic self-expectations. They are impulsive and anxious; are arrogant, envious, and lacking in empathy; have ideas of omnipotence and of being "a special person"; become quickly dissatisfied with others; and maintain superficial, exploitative interpersonal relationships. Under stress and when others are not adequately admiring, they may become depressed, develop somatic complaints, have brief psychotic episodes, or display extreme rage. Mixtures with other personality disorders are common. Long-term psychotherapy helps.

ANXIOUS FEARFUL CLUSTER

AVOIDANT PERSONALITY DISORDER (DSM-IV p. 662, 301.82)

The classic presentation is of an exceedingly shy, lonely, hypersensitive individual with low self-esteem who would rather avoid personal contact than face any potential social disapproval, even though desperate for interpersonal involvement (as opposed to the schizoid person). They assume others will be critical: This affects performance in school, work, and life. These patients are troubled by anxiety (especially social phobia) and depression. Group therapy may help (9).

DEPENDENT PERSONALITY DISORDER (DSM-IV p. 665, 301.6)

These are excessively passive, unsure, pessimistic, isolated people who are hypersensitive to criticism and who become abnormally dependent on one or more people. Initially acceptable, the behavior can become subtly controlling of others. Anxiety and depression are common, particularly if the dependent relationship is threatened.

OBSESSIVE-COMPULSIVE PERSONALITY DISORDER
(DSM-IV p. 669, 301.4)

These patients, frequently successful men (M:F = 2:1), are inhibited, stubborn, perfectionistic, judgmental, overly conscientious, rigid, and chronically anxious individuals who avoid intimacy and experience little pleasure from life. They are indecisive yet demanding and are often perceived as cold and reserved. They are at risk to develop depression and *perhaps* OCD. Psychotherapy can effect changes over time.

ATTENTION-DEFICIT/HYPERACTIVITY DISORDER
(DSM-IV p. 78, 314.01)

Attention-deficit/hyperactivity disorder (ADHD) is a disorder of early childhood that can continue to produce problems well into adulthood (10,11) and has many features of, and is frequently mistaken for, a personality disorder. These patients have been distractible, *disorganized,* inattentive, *impulsive,* unable to tolerate stress, restless, quick tempered, and display *affective lability* (often hour by hour) since childhood. They may have learning disabilities. Their lability impairs interpersonal relations and job stability and often produces depression. They are at serious risk for drug abuse and alcoholism (12). Frequently, with age, the full criteria cannot be met (usually the hyperactivity disappears) and the diagnosis becomes *ADHD, In Partial Remission.* Differentiate from personality disorders, cyclothymic disorder (more recent onset), intermittent explosive disorder (normal between episodes), and primary depression. ADHD is most effectively treated with stimulants (e.g., methylphenidate 10 mg PO tid to six times a day), but use them very cautiously due to abuse potential. [Propranolol, the TCAs (13), and bupropion may be alternatives.] Combine with supportive psychotherapy.

REFERENCES

1. Millon T. *Disorders of personality: DSM-IV and beyond.* New York: Wiley, 1996.
2. McGuffin P, Thapar A. The genetics of personality disorder. *Br J Psychiatry* 1992;160:12–23.
3. Livesley WJ, Jang KL, Vernon PA. Phenotypic and genetic structure of traits delineating personality disorder. *Arch Gen Psychiatry* 1998;55: 941–948.
4. Stone MH. Long-term outcome in personality disorders. *Br J Psychiatry* 1993;162:299–313.
5. Davis JM, Janicak PG, Ayd FJ. Psychopharmacotherapy of the personality-disordered patient. *Psychiatric Ann* 1995;25:614–620.
6. Lencz T, Raine A, Scerbo A, et al. Impaired eye tracking in undergraduates with schizotypal personality disorder. *Am J Psychiatry* 1993; 150:152–154.
7. Voglmaier MM, Seidman LJ, Salisbury D, et al. Neuropsychological dysfunction in schizotypal personality disorder. *Biol Psychiatry* 1997; 41:530–540.
8. Widiger RA, Cadoret R, Hare R, et al. DSM-IV antisocial personality disorder field trial. *J Abnorm Psychol* 1996;105:3–16.
9. Alden L. Short-term structured treatment for avoidant personality disorder. *J Consult Clin Psychol* 1989;57:756–764.
10. Wender PH. Attention-deficit hyperactivity disorder in adults. *Psychiatr Clin North Am* 1998;21:761–774.
11. Toone BK, van der Linden GJH. Attention deficit hyperactivity disorder or hyperkinetic disorder in adults. *Br J Psychiatry* 1997;170: 489–491.

12. Mannuzza S, Klein RG, Bessler A, et al. Adult psychiatric status of hyperactive boys grown up. *Am J Psychiatry* 1998;155:493–498.
13. Wilens TE, Biederman J, Prince J, et al. Six-week, double-blind, placebo-controlled study of desipramine for adult attention deficit hyperactivity disorder. *Am J Psychiatry* 1996;153:1147–1153.

Chapter 21

Mental Retardation

There are 2–4 million mentally retarded persons in the U.S. [1%–2% or more of population, depending on upper cutoff; M:F = 1.5:1; coded on Axis II in (DSM-IV)] of whom 80%–85% are only mildly retarded (1). The diagnosis of *mental retardation* requires decreased intellectual functioning (measured by standard IQ tests—two standard deviations below the mean IQ of 100) *and* impaired general functioning. Its presentation is modified by age, experience, and the environmental and cultural setting. It is most commonly first identified in grade-school children, and the prevalence peaks at age 15 years. [Most mildly retarded *adults,* when no longer in school, are indistinguishable from the lowest socioeconomic segment of the general population and may no longer receive the diagnosis of mental retardation—i.e., they develop skills, adapt, and "grow out of it" (2), but, although self-sufficient, they tend to be poor and experience stress and emotional problems (3).] Adults with intellectual impairment that developed before age 18 have (usually nonprogressive) **retardation,** and those developing it after age 18 have **dementia.**

CLASSIFICATION

- **MILD MENTAL RETARDATION** (DSM-IV p. 41, 317)—IQ 50–70; considered "*educable.*" Usually recognized when they enter school (and are tested) and require special education. Constitutes **85%** of the retarded (but *this* is the group that decreases markedly with adulthood). Most become self-supporting, with help, although they have limited judgment, social sensitivity, and insight.

- **MODERATE MENTAL RETARDATION** (DSM-IV p. 41, 318.0)—IQ 35–50; *10%* of all retarded. Usually recognized during preschool years. They are "*trainable*," can learn simple work skills, can read at a 2nd grade level and speak simply, and can be partly self-supporting in sheltered settings. They tend to be clumsy and uncoordinated.
- **SEVERE MENTAL RETARDATION** (DSM-IV p. 41, 318.1)— IQ 20–35; *3%–4%* of all retarded. These are the *dependent retarded:* They are capable of the most simple speech but require institutional or other intensely supportive care. Malformations and severe physical handicaps are frequent.
- **PROFOUND MENTAL RETARDATION** (DSM-IV p. 41, 318.2)—IQ below 20; *1%* of all retarded. They are totally dependent on others for survival and usually have significant neurologic damage; cannot walk or talk.

A presumably retarded patient who is untestable is considered to have **MENTAL RETARDATION, SEVERITY UNSPECIFIED** (DSM-IV p. 42, 319).

CAUSES

Distinct causes (usually biologic) are identified in less than 50% of patients; these are most of the moderately-to-profoundly retarded patients. Other causes include environmental factors (e.g., pre- and perinatal problems, infant illness, *psychosocial neglect,* malnutrition), with an uncertain polygenic contribution in some cases. Moderate-to-profound retardation is distributed uniformly across social classes, whereas mild retardation (usually from sociocultural etiology) is weighted toward the lower classes. Retardation is a familial disorder (genetics and/or environment); the risk of retardation in a child with normal parents and siblings is less than *2%*, whereas the risk if both parents and one sibling are afflicted may be as great as *40%–70%* (4).

Biological causes include

- Chromosomal abnormalities—Numerous types including *Down's syndrome* (5) [mongolism, trisomy 21; the *most* common abnormality; more typical among older mothers; 10%–16% of all retarded; most develop *Alzheimer's disease* in their

30s or 40s (6)], *fragile X syndrome* (7) (2%–7% of retardation among males; 1 in 2,000 live births; *second* most common abnormality), Klinefelter's syndrome (XXY; 1%–2% of retarded), Cri-du-chat syndrome, and Turner's syndrome (XO/XX).

- Dominant genetic inheritance—Neurofibromatosis (Von Recklinghausen's disease), Huntington's chorea (with childhood onset), Sturge-Weber syndrome, tuberous sclerosis.
- Metabolic disorders—Phenylketonuria (PKU) (early detection essential), Hartnup disease, fructose intolerance, galactosemia, Wilson's disease, a variety of lipid disorders, hypothyroidism, hypoglycemia.
- Prenatal disorders—Maternal rubella (particularly in the 1st trimester), syphilis, toxoplasmosis, or diabetes; maternal alcohol abuse [fetal alcohol syndrome (8)] and use of some drugs (e.g., thalidomide); toxemia of pregnancy; erythroblastosis fetalis; maternal malnutrition.
- Birth trauma—Difficult delivery with physical trauma and/or anoxia, prematurity.
- Brain trauma—Tumors, infection (particularly encephalitis, neonatal meningitis), accidents, toxins (e.g., **lead**, mercury), hydrocephalus, numerous types of cranial abnormalities.

Social causes produce *most of the mild retardation* and include substandard education, environmental deprivation, childhood abuse and neglect, and restricted activity.

Rule out pervasive developmental disorders, dementia, and residual schizophrenia. Rule out **BORDERLINE INTELLECTUAL FUNCTIONING** (DSM-IV p. 684, V62.89; IQ 70–85). Look for associated psychiatric or neurologic syndromes.

TREATMENT AND PROGNOSIS

Formal cognitive testing at 1–2 years of age often is predictive of global outcome in many cases (9). However, mildly retarded individuals do develop further, often at an unpredictable but slower rate, with education (particularly with careful *mainstreaming*) and a supportive environment. They are at risk for adjustment reaction, hyperactivity, and depression [50% or so present with aggression and self-injury (10), psychotic reactions, and behavioral disturbances 2° to a negative self-image at some time].

Treat the patient with supportive reality-oriented psychotherapy. Determine the patient's coping style and temperamental strengths and encourage them but do not demand too much (11). Simple behavior modification techniques may be very effective and should be part of any treatment program.

Severely retarded persons may require some form of institutionalization, yet training in sheltered settings should be considered if possible. If the patient lives with her family, treat the family. Parents and siblings frequently display anger, rejection, overprotection and overcontrol, denial, and/or guilt—all of which should be recognized and dealt with by the physician. Provide genetic counseling. Coordinate with outside agencies and specialists, when available.

Psychiatric syndromes are 3–4 times more common among the retarded. Consider psychopharmacology in patients with typical syndromes (12). Low doses of minor or major tranquilizers may help behavior problems (e.g., aggressiveness): don't overuse (it is easy to do). Lithium or propranolol may moderate self-abuse and aggression in some cases.

REFERENCES

1. Burack JA, Hodapp RM, Zigler E. *Handbook of mental retardation and development.* New York: Cambridge University Press, 1998.
2. Torrey WC. Psychiatric care of adults with developmental disabilities and mental illness in the community. *Community Ment Health J* 1993; 29:461–481.
3. Maughan B, Collishaw S, Pickles A. Mild mental retardation: psychosocial functioning in adulthood. *Psychol Med* 1999;29:351–366.
4. Thapar A, Gottesman II, Owen MJ, et al. The genetics of mental retardation. *Br J Psychiatry* 1994;164:747–758.
5. Hayes A, Batshaw ML. Down's syndrome. *Pediatr Clin North Am* 1993; 40:523–535.
6. Holland AJ, Oliver C. Down's syndrome and the links with Alzheimer's disease. *J Neurol Neurosurg Psychiatry* 1995;59:111–114.
7. Turk J. Fragile X syndrome. *Arch Dis Childhood* 1995;72:3–5.
8. Streissguth A. *Fetal alcohol syndrome.* Baltimore, MD: Paul H. Brooks Publishing Co., 1997.
9. Largo RH, Graf S, Kundu S, et al. Predicting developmental outcome at school age from infant tests of normal, at-risk and retarded infants. *Dev Med Child Neurol* 1990;32:30–45.
10. Charlot LR. Irritability, aggression, and depression in adults with mental retardation. *Psychiatric Ann* 1997;27:190–197.

11. Siperstein GN, Leffert JS. Comparison of socially accepted and rejected children with mental retardation. *Am J Ment Retard* 1997; 101:339–351.
12. Boshes RA. Pharmacotherapy for patients with mental retardation and mental illness. *Psychiatric Ann* 1987;17:627–632.

Chapter 22

The Psychotherapies

There are dozens of different psychotherapies addressing innumerable different patient problems (1). With the possible exception of a few specific behavioral and cognitive-behavioral methods applied to several discrete problems, rigorous proof of psychotherapy's effectiveness does not exist. However, there is much nonrigorous but very compelling experience indicating that various psychotherapies can help many patients; almost every therapist educates, gets patients to voice their concerns, encourages them to try out new behaviors, etc. Unfortunately, specific indications for specific therapies generally are not available. Some experts argue that many supposedly different psychotherapeutic methods are actually quite similar in practice (2). Other experts suggest that trained therapists utilizing specific techniques may be less important for the patient's improvement than the therapist's personal characteristics of *accurate empathy, nonpossessive warmth,* and *genuineness.* Studies comparing the effectiveness of empathic trainees to experienced therapists have often found only modest differences in outcome (3).

Psychotherapy is a field without a high level of scientific objectivity. However, it is clear that some patients benefit from such care and that an essential ingredient to that care is a good patient–therapist relationship built on trust and genuine interest. Psychotherapy is an art, and a good therapist does make a difference. In general, you need to find a therapy that is a "good fit" for the patient (i.e., the patient is comfortable with the therapist and the type of therapy). Patients resist psychotherapy unless they feel that it is both tolerable and likely to be of benefit; the drop-out rate from therapy can be quite high. Individual treatment is the most common form of psychotherapy and comes in endless variations; group, family, and marital therapy are in widespread use as well (4).

INDIVIDUAL THERAPY

Supportive Therapy

This is probably the most common form of individual therapy (5). Therapists skilled in this method include psychiatrists, clinical psychologists, and social workers, although some approximation of supportive therapy is used by just about anyone who tries to help a person in emotional distress. The goal is to evaluate the patient's current life situation and strengths and weaknesses and then to help him or her make whatever realistic changes will allow them to be more functional. Patients usually are seen weekly (or more often) for several weeks or months (although some patients are followed infrequently for years). Also included is brief (1–3 sessions) crisis intervention.

The therapist deals with the patient's symptoms but works very little with the patient's unconscious processes and does not attempt major personality change. Psychological defenses are reinforced, and techniques used include *reassurance,* suggestion, ventilation, abreaction, and environmental manipulation. The therapist must be active, interested, empathic, and warm—listen to the patient, understand concerns, and help him or her find direction. Medication may be used.

Patients who are failing to cope successfully with present stress are good candidates, whether or not they have underlying psychiatric problems. Patients with serious psychiatric illnesses (e.g., schizophrenia, major affective disorder) often benefit from concurrent use of biologic methods and supportive psychotherapy.

Psychoanalytic Psychotherapy

Psychoanalysis is the classic, long-term, insight-oriented therapy. The goal is to make major personality changes by identifying and modifying ("working through") unconscious conflicts by means of free association, analysis of transference and resistance, and dream interpretation. An "analysis" typically takes several hundred hours.

"Neurotics" and those with personality disorders are the preferred patients. It is lengthy, expensive, and of uncertain effectiveness and so is infrequently used.

Psychoanalytic psychotherapy is similar to supportive therapy in that the goal is removal of symptoms yet is similar to psychoanalysis in requiring a dynamic understanding of the patient's unconscious conflicts (insight) and in utilizing analysis of the transference and dream interpretation. It is briefer than psychoanalysis and used much more often.

Recently, *brief psychotherapy* has been explored as a way to have an impact on a patient's problems while at the same time limiting both the number of therapy sessions (12–25 or more) and the number of issues addressed. Usually, a single conflict or interpersonal issue is chosen for therapy and explored in depth, most commonly from a psychodynamic perspective. Early results appear promising (6). Recognize that brief therapy can be approached from numerous different theoretical perspectives as well, for example, using *humanistic principles* such as a belief that we all share an innate need for acceptance, love, and respect and that given proper support and help we all have an innate drive toward psychological growth and health.

Interpersonal Therapy

A recent, reasonably well-controlled study (the New Haven-Boston Collaborative Depression Project) compared the effectiveness of various forms of psychotherapy with, and without, medication in the treatment of mild to moderate depression (7,8). *Interpersonal therapy* (ITP) was found effective. The combination of ITP and drugs improved most depressions and maintenance medication and/or ITP seemed to prevent relapse.

ITP focuses on the patient's interpersonal relationships, their nature and their failings, and on improving those relationships. The idea is that if a person has vigorous, healthy, rewarding relations with other people, they are less likely to become, be, or stay depressed (or anxious, etc.) and they are more likely to be happy. Evidence suggests this to be true. Treatment consists of

1. *Education* (e.g., about depression; how common it is, its biologic nature, the risk that we all share of becoming depressed under stress, etc.). The effort is made to *destigmatize* the patient's mental problem.

2. *Information collection* about the patient's interpersonal relationships in an effort to determine which one(s) is not working. Such an inventory of the important interpersonal relationships in a person's life usually identifies, interestingly enough, a relationship that is poor or failing. Treatment begins with concentration on that relationship.

3. There are several classic types of problems within relationships. Identify the most important one present and attempt to repair it. Sample problems include
   - **Interpersonal role disputes:** Is the patient "hopelessly" at odds with someone of vital importance to him or her (e.g., spouse, parent, child, boss, etc.)? SOLUTION: you help the patient (a) determine what the dispute is about so he or she can see *both* sides, (b) clarify his or her own position in the dispute and also bring a degree of objectivity to his or her view of the problem, (c) form a reasonable plan of action to resolve the dispute, (d) identify any ways in which he or she may have been *miscommunicating with* or *misperceiving* the other person, and (e) modify expectations for the relationship, if they seem unrealistic.
   - **Role transitions:** Has a change in a relationship already occurred and is the patient failing to cope with the new situation? SOLUTION: there is "mourning" going on here too—grieving over a loss of an old role—and you need to help facilitate that mourning as well and encourage the patient to see this new life situation as positive and as a "growth opportunity."
   - **Grief and loss:** Has a relationship been lost and the patient been grieving? SOLUTION: (a) you facilitate the mourning process and (b) help the patient reestablish interests and develop new relationships to substitute for that which was lost.

4. This is meant to be *brief* therapy, lasting no more than 12 sessions of about 1 hour each. (That worked in the depression study.)

Cognitive-Behavioral Therapy

Cognitive-behavioral therapy (9,10) is a mixture of cognitive therapy and behavior therapy. It attributes emotional difficulties to faulty thinking or beliefs (**cognition**) that lead to counterproductive

behavior. Psychiatric conditions presumably improve when the patient's thinking is more accurate and when the behavior is more appropriate. Thus, the therapist works with the patient to identify and correct misperceptions (one by one) and (mis)behaviors. Therapy is very reality based and emphasizes the "here and now" (what is the patient thinking now; how is the patient behaving now). The patient is encouraged to think about his thinking. Cognitive-behavioral therapy has been used most successfully in the treatment of mild-to-moderate depression, panic disorder, OCD, and eating disorders but seems to be even more widely useful.

Behavior Therapy

Behavior therapy is based on *learning theory,* which postulates that problem behaviors (i.e., almost any of the manifestations of psychiatric conditions) are involuntarily acquired due to inappropriate learning. Therapy concentrates on changing *behavior* (behavior modification) rather than on changing unconscious or conscious thought patterns, and to that end it is very directive (i.e., patient receives much instruction and direction). Specific techniques to facilitate those changes include the following:

- **Operant conditioning**—These therapeutic techniques are based on careful evaluation and modification of the antecedents and consequences of a patient's behavior. Desired behavior is encouraged by *positive reinforcement* and discouraged by *negative reinforcement.* These new ways of responding to the patient can be taught to the people who live with the patient or, for inpatients, may take the form of a *token economy.*
- **Aversion therapy**—A patient is given an unpleasant aversive stimulus (e.g., electric shock, loud sound) when his or her behavior is undesirable. Some of these procedures have been legally discouraged. An alternate technique, *covert sensitization,* is less objectionable because it uses unpleasant thoughts as the aversive stimulus.
- **Implosive therapy**—The patient with a situation-caused anxiety is directly exposed for a length of time to that situation (*flooding*) or exposed in imagination (*implosion*).
- **Systematic desensitization**—The anxious or phobic patient is exposed to a gradual hierarchy of frightening situations or

objects, beginning with the least worrisome. The patient eventually learns to handle the more frightening ones. If this is paired with relaxation (i.e., an antagonistic response pattern—relaxation is incompatible with anxiety), the technique is *reciprocal inhibition.*

Common to these methods (and numerous others) is rigorous data collection. Behavior therapy relies on careful measurement of behavior. A technique is considered useful only if it is successful, and its success is determined by whether it eliminates measurable undesired behavior or increases desired behavior.

Cognitive Therapy

1. The way a person interprets her life experiences on a day-to-day basis determines how she feels day in and day out.
2. People with emotional distress tend to interpret their experiences in a dysfunctional, distorted way: these become the **core beliefs** of the person.
3. Over time, these distortions become "habitual errors in thinking." Common logical errors include, among others, *overgeneralization* (generalizes from a single event to all situations, e.g., if something went wrong once, a similar event is likely to go equally wrong), *magnification* (blowing an event out of proportion), *selective abstraction* (drawing conclusions from a detail taken out of context), and *personalization* (relating an event to yourself when there is no reason to do so).
4. Layered on top of these dysfunctional core beliefs and logical errors are **automatic thoughts**. These are "reflex thoughts" that we have in many situations; they are quick and we are barely aware of them, yet they determine to a large extent how we react emotionally to events. Automatic thoughts are typically followed by emotions such as sadness, anxiety, or anger.
5. Treatment involves identifying the core beliefs, habitual errors in thinking, and automatic thoughts and correcting them.

Cognitive therapy has been shown to be effective for a number of common psychiatric conditions, particularly depression, panic disorder, and generalized anxiety disorder. There is sufficient, double-blind evidence that cognitive therapy really works, particularly when coupled with behavioral approaches.

GROUP THERAPY

Group therapy (11) comes in many different forms, most derived from types of individual therapy.

- **Interpersonal exploration groups**—The goal is to develop self-awareness of interpersonal styles through corrective feedback from other group members. The patient is accepted and supported, thus promoting self-esteem. It is the most common type of group therapy.
- **Guidance-inspirational groups**—Highly structured, cohesive, supportive groups that minimize the importance of insight and maximize the value of ventilation and camaraderie. Groups may be large (e.g., Alcoholics Anonymous). Members often are chosen because they "have the same problem."
- **Psychoanalytically oriented therapy**—A loosely structured group technique in which the therapist makes interpretations about a patient's unconscious conflicts and processes from observed group interactions.

Numerous other types of group therapies include behavioral therapy, Gestalt, encounter, psychodrama, transactional analysis (TA), marathon, est, etc.

Groups may run for weeks, months, or years, and usually meet weekly. They usually have 5–12 members (depending on type). Therapists from many different disciplines conduct groups; many groups run with cotherapists.

Some groups have patients with only one diagnosis (e.g., schizophrenia, alcoholism), whereas others are mixed. It is not clear which patients will benefit (or will be harmed) by group therapy, but most patients can be treated safely in groups. Most of the success of a group appears to depend more on the experience, sensitivity, warmth, and charisma of the leader than on the group's theoretical orientation.

A group experience that is too intense or confrontative can produce anxiety, depression, or psychotic reactions in susceptible patients. Acutely psychotic patients should not be included, and paranoid individuals make poor group members.

FAMILY THERAPY

Family therapy (12) can be conceptualized as a variant of group therapy. There are numerous types of family therapy but no "one right way." Although a family often enters therapy because one of the family members is "having problems," it is the implicit or explicit assumption of many family therapists that the family system is sick, not the patient. The expectation is that improvement in unhealthy interpersonal interactions and communications will result in improvement of the identified patient.

Most (but not all) family therapists recognize that some patients bring problems to family therapy that are not due to family malfunctioning, but most therapists argue that those problems are frequently worsened by any untreated malfunctioning.

MARITAL THERAPY

Therapy of a married couple is often called for if that relationship is at risk. It is particularly common if there is a psychosexual problem present. Theoretic orientations and treatment techniques are diverse; none has been clearly shown to be superior. There are no clear guidelines for choosing couples likely to improve with marital therapy. Therapists may come from one of several professional disciplines (e.g., psychiatry, psychology, social work, marriage and family counseling).

MILIEU THERAPY

Milieu therapy usually takes place in an inpatient "therapeutic community." Often the entire community is geared toward support for the patient and toward helping that patient develop more adaptive coping skills. In a sense, all the staff members are therapists and all the patients are likewise concerned with facilitating each other's well-being. It is a useful adjunct to other forms of therapy (e.g., pharmacotherapy).

REFERENCES

1. Tillett R. Psychotherapy assessment and treatment selection. *Br J Psychiatry* 1996;168:10–15.
2. Kovitz B. To a beginning psychotherapist: how to conduct individual psychotherapy. *Am J Psychother* 1998;52:103–115.
3. Krupnick JL, Sotsky SM, Simmens S, et al. The role of the therapeutic alliance in psychotherapy and pharmacotherapy outcome. *J Consult Clin Psychol* 1996;64:532–539.

4. Gabbard GO, Lazar SG, Hornberger J, et al. The economic impact of psychotherapy: a review. *Am J Psychiatry* 1997;154:147–155.

5. Rockland LH. A review of supportive psychotherapy, 1986–1992. *Hosp Commun Psychiatry* 1993;44:1053–1060.

6. Levenson H. *Time-limited dynamic psychotherapy: a guide to clinical practice.* New York: Basic Books, 1995.

7. Elkin I, Shea T, Watkins JT, et al. NIMH treatment of depression collaborative research program. *Arch Gen Psychiatry* 1989;46:971–982.

8. Elkin I, Gibbons RD, Shea MT, et al. Science is not a trial (but it can sometimes be a tribulation). *J Consult Clin Psychol* 1996;64:92–103.

9. Beck AT. *Cognitive therapy and the emotional disorders.* New York: Intern University Press, 1976.

10. Beck AT, Emery G. *Anxiety disorders and phobias: a cognitive perspective.* New York: Basic Books, 1985.

11. Yalom ID. *The theory and practice of group psychotherapy.* New York: Basic Books, 1995.

12. Pittman FS. *Turning points: treating families in transition and crisis.* New York: Norton, 1987.

Chapter 23

Biologic Therapy

ANTIPSYCHOTICS

These are the "major tranquilizers" that revolutionized psychiatry by providing an effective treatment for large numbers of psychotic patients. Their antipsychotic effect is not due to sedation but to a specific action on the thought and mood disorder.

Drugs Available

Many different antipsychotics are available and are divided into two major categories: for the first 30 years, the *traditional antipsychotics* were used, drugs that acted through powerful D_2 receptor blockade, and since the early 1990s, *atypical antipsychotics* have been added, drugs that affect the D_2 receptor to a lesser degree while providing significant blockade of the $5\text{-}HT_{2A}$ receptor (1,2). Although both types of drugs are effective, the newer medication has several significant advantages that rapidly have caused them to become the "class of choice." Common examples of both classes are listed in Table 23.1.

Traditional Antipsychotics

Indications for Use

Recommended for:

1. Acute schizophrenia and other acute psychoses (e.g., amphetamine psychosis, organic psychoses). Should be used in

TABLE 23.1 Antipsychotics

	Equivalent doses (mg)
Traditional antipsychotics	
Phenothiazines	
Dimethylamino-alkyl derivatives	
chlorpromazine (Thorazine)	100
Piperidine-alkyl derivatives	
thioridazine (Mellaril)	100
mesoridazine (Serentil)	50
Piperazine-alkyl derivatives	
fluphenazine (Prolixin)	1–2
fluphenazine decanoate (long-acting)	
trifluoperazine (Stelazine)	8
perphenazine (Trilafon)	10
Thioxanthenes	
thiothixene (Navane)	4
Dibenzoxazepines	
loxapine (Loxitane)	15
Dihydroindolones	
molindone (Moban)	15
Butyrophenones	
haloperidol (Haldol)	1–2
haloperidol decanoate (long acting)	
Diphenylbutylpiperidines	
pimozide (Orap)	1–2

	Therapeutic dose (mg/day)
Atypical antipsychotics	
clozapine (Clozaril)	100–900
olanzapine (Zyprexa)	10–25
quetiapine fumarate (Seroquel)	100–750
risperidone (Risperdal)	4–6
ziprasidone (Zeldox)	40–160

    conjunction with lithium in the acute manic attacks of bipolar disorder.

2. Chronic schizophrenia.
3. Major depression with significant psychotic features—used in conjunction with an antidepressant.
4. Tourette's syndrome—haloperidol is the drug most commonly used.

Other uses:

- Antipsychotics can also be of temporary use in several other conditions (e.g., acute agitation of a nonpsychotic nature, antiemesis, etc.).

Mechanisms of Action

The dopamine hypothesis postulates that schizophrenia is secondary to increased central dopamine activity. Traditional antipsychotics are believed to act primarily by a broad and powerful postsynaptic blockade of the D_2 receptors. The three major central nervous system (CNS) dopamine pathways affected by these medications, with their putative activities are:

Nigrostriatal—extrapyramidal actions
Tuberoinfundibular—endocrine actions (increased prolactin)
Mesolimbic—antipsychotic actions (probably)

The different side-effect patterns of the various antipsychotic drugs are believed to be due to their different locations of primary activity. However, traditional antipsychotics also block central noradrenergic (NE) receptors; thus, we cannot be certain whether DA or NE blockage (or another mechanism entirely) is responsible for the antipsychotic effect of these drugs.

Pharmacokinetics

Chlorpromazine (as a classic example) is variably absorbed from the intestine and is probably partly degraded in the mucosal wall. It is approximately 95% protein bound. Much higher blood levels are attained after IM or IV than PO administration. The half-life is 1–2 or more days but variable, with most of the drug stored in body fat. There are *marked* interindividual differences in blood levels (reasons are unclear).

Metabolism is complex (e.g., chlorpromazine is degraded by sulfoxidation, hydroxylation, deamination, demethylation, etc., to form well over 100 metabolites). Some metabolites are active, some inactive; not completely worked out. In part because of this complexity, measured plasma levels of many antipsychotics are not clinically useful. In contrast, certain other antipsychotics (e.g., haloperidol, thiothixene) have a simple metabolism; however, their plasma measurement as a guide to outcome is of uncertain value.

Side Effects

Side effects are common and are almost unavoidable at higher drug dosages. Fewer side-effect problems is one of the major reasons for the superiority of the newer antipsychotics. The particular pattern of side effects is in part determined by the chemical class of any given antipsychotic.

These side effects also have marked interindividual variability. The most common side effects of these medications include (Table 23.2) sedation, extrapyramidal and anticholinergic symptoms, hypotension, weight gain, and reduced libido, but many other side effects occur as well.

TABLE 23.2   Most Common Side Effects of the Traditional Antipsychotics

Drug	Sedation	Extrapyramidal	Hypotension
Phenothiazines			
Aliphatic	3 +	2 +	3 +
Piperidine	2 +	1 +	2 +
Piperazine	1 +	3 +	1 +
Dibenzoxazepines	2 +	3 +	2 +
Butyrophenones	2 +	3 +	1 +
Dihydroindolones	1 +	2 +	1 +

Sedation: Common; use a QD schedule, if possible
Anticholinergic symptoms:

- *Dry mouth*—Common. May lead to moniliasis, parotitis, and an increase in cavities. Consider treatment with oral water and ice, sugarless gum; also neostigmine 7.5–15 mg PO, pilocarpine 2.5 mg PO qid, or bethanechol 75 mg daily.
- *Constipation*—Treat with stool softeners.
- *Blurred vision*—Near vision. Treat with physostigmine drops, 0.25% solution, 1 drop q6 hr, if a major problem.
- Urinary hesitancy and retention—Consider using Urecholine 10–25 mg PO tid.
- Exacerbation of glaucoma.
- **Central anticholinergic syndrome**—Occurs particularly in those patients simultaneously taking several drugs with anticholinergic properties (e.g., an OD or a patient taking an antipsychotic, an antidepressant, and an antiparkinsonian). The syndrome can vary from mild anxiety and vasodilatation to a toxic delirium or even coma. It is much more common in the elderly. Symptoms and signs to be looked for include:
  - Anxiety, restlessness, agitation—grading into confusion, incoherence, disorientation, memory impairment, visual and auditory hallucinations—grading into seizures, stupor, and coma.

- **Warm and dry skin,** flushed face, dry mouth, hyperpyrexia.
- Blurred vision, dilated pupils.
- Absent bowel sounds.

Treat an acute delirium with withdrawal of the causative agent, close medical supervision (e.g., cardiac monitor), and physostigmine 1–2 mg IM or slowly IV (e.g., 1 mg/min). Repeat in 15–30 minutes and then every 1–2 hours, if needed. Avoid physostigmine in patients with bowel or bladder obstruction, peptic ulcer, asthma, glaucoma, heart disease, diabetes, or hypothyroidism. Watch for cholinergic over-dosage (salivation, sweating, etc.) and treat with atropine (0.5 mg for each mg of physostigmine).

Extrapyramidal symptoms: Common, get worse with stress, disappear during sleep, and wax and wane over time.
- *Acute dystonic reaction*—An involuntary sustained contraction of a skeletal muscle that usually appears suddenly (over 5–60 minutes). The jaw muscles are most frequently involved (i.e., "lockjaw") but other muscle systems may also be disturbed (e.g., torticollis, carpopedal spasm, oculogyric crisis, even opisthotonos). Usually occurs during the first 2 days of treatment (in 2%–10% of patients—more common in younger patients).
- *Parkinson-like syndrome*—The three primary symptoms occur individually or together, usually during weeks 1–4 of treatment. They are more common in older patients.
  "Tremor"—An irregular tremor of the upper extremities, tongue, and jaw. It occurs with both movement and rest and is slower than the tremors produced by TCAs and lithium.
  "Rigidity"—A cogwheel rigidity that starts with the shoulders and spreads to the upper extremities and then throughout the body.
  "Akinesia"—A "zombielike" effect with slowness, fatigue, micrographia, and little facial expression. It may occur alone and at any time during the course of treatment and is easily mistaken for social withdrawal or depression.
- *Akathisia:* Common. Patients are fidgety, constantly move their hands and feet, rock from the waist, and shift from foot to foot. Easily mistaken for anxiety or agitation. The patients are typically dysphoric. Treat with anticholinergics, propranolol (10 mg tid, 30–120 mg/day), or lorazepam.

- Rabbit syndrome: Involuntary chewing movements.
- **Tardive dyskinesia:** Slow choreiform or tic-like movements, usually of the tongue and facial muscles but occasionally of the upper extremities or the whole body. Risk is increased in the aged, those with OBS, females, high doses of medication, simultaneous use of several antipsychotics, and possibly long duration of treatment. Develops over months or years of antipsychotic use, a few severe cases may be irreversible, but it usually follows a stable, benign, long-term course. Symptoms disappear with an increased dosage of antipsychotic: Do not "misread" the movements as a worsening psychosis, raise the dose of medication, remove the symptom, and thus begin a vicious cycle. "Drug holidays" do not seem to prevent, and may even worsen, the development of tardive dyskinesia. There is no acceptable treatment. Try to discontinue the antipsychotic, if possible.

Treatment of extrapyramidal symptoms:

Treat with the anticholinergic *antiparkinsonism drugs* (Table 23.3). Begin at a lower dosage and raise over several days. Use for several weeks, then discontinue if possible. Try not to use for more than 2–3 months (although they may be necessary long term in a few patients). They probably should not be used prophylactically (begun when antipsychotics are started) except in those patients very likely to be resistant to taking medications. Treat acute dystonic reactions immediately (IM or IV) with (e.g.) Cogentin 1 mg, Benadryl 25–50 mg, or Valium 5–10 mg – then begin regular oral dose for several weeks. These drugs often worsen symptoms of TD; they may also be abused.

TABLE 23.3   Antiparkinsonism Drugs

Drug	Typical dosage
Benztropine (Cogentin)	1–4 mg, q.d.–b.i.d., p.o.
Biperiden (Akineton)	1–2 mg, t.i.d., q.i.d., p.o.
Procyclidine (Kemadrin)	2–5 mg, t.i.d.–q.i.d., p.o.
Trihexyphenidyl (Artane, Tremin)	2–5 mg, t.i.d.–q.i.d., p.o.
Diphenhydramine (Benadryl)	25–50 mg, t.i.d.–q.i.d., p.o.
Amantadine (Symmetral)	100 mg, q.d.–t.i.d., p.o.

α-Adrenergic blocking symptoms: Orthostatic hypotension, inhibition of ejaculation (particularly thioridazine).

Cholestatic jaundice: Probably a sensitivity reaction. Fever and eosinophilia, usually during the first 2 months of treatment (in

1% of patients taking chlorpromazine). Little cross-sensitivity with other antipsychotics.

Agranulocytosis: Usually in elderly females during the first 4 months of treatment but can occur anytime. Train patients to report persistent sore throats, infections, or fever. Rare.

Neuroleptic malignant syndrome (NMS): Rapidly developing (hours to 1–2 days) muscular rigidity and cogwheeling, fever, confusion, hypertension, sweating, tachycardia. Look for rhabdomyolysis with myoglobinemia and *very* elevated CPK. In 1% or more of patients, particularly (but not exclusively) after high-dose, high-potency depot medications. Often fatal if untreated. Stop medications immediately; provide medical support; consider treatment with dantrolene (muscle relaxant; 400 mg/day) and bromocriptine (dopamine agonist; 7.5–45 mg/day, tid). Patient may recover over 5–15 days. It typically does *not* recur upon later reexposure to antipsychotics.

Hypothermia; hyperthermia: Watch out for hot seclusion rooms.

Weight gain, obesity.

Pigmentary changes in skin: Particularly with chlorpromazine. A tan, gray, or blue color.

Retinitis pigmentosa—Possible blindness. Occurs with dosages of thioridazine greater than 800 mg/day.

Photosensitivity: Bad sunburns with Thorazine.

Grand mal seizures: Particularly with rapid increases in dose.

Nonspecific skin rashes: In 5%.

Reduced libido in males and females.

Increased prolactin levels: Produces galactorrhea, amenorrhea, and lactation.

ECG changes: Particularly with thioridazine—T-wave inversions, occasionally arrhythmias.

Appears safe during pregnancy: no known congenital abnormalities. Slight hypertonicity among newborns, but little effect on nursing infant.

Suicide is difficult but possible with the antipsychotics—requires very large doses.

Drug Interactions

Antacids may inhibit absorption of oral antipsychotics. TCAs and SSRIs may inhibit antipsychotic metabolism and raise plasma levels, and vice versa.

Treatment Principles

- *Drug choice:* The primary reason to choose one drug over another is the side-effect spectrum; each medication is equally capable of controlling psychosis when used appropriately. If a patient or a similarly affected family member has responded well to one medication, try it. If a patient has a seizure disorder, use a high-potency drug (e.g., fluphenazine, haloperidol).

- *Treatment of acute psychosis:* Sedating antipsychotics that can be given IM usually provide the best control initially (e.g., haloperidol, chlorpromazine), although they have no long-term advantages. Give orally if the patient is cooperative, IM if not.

  1. If possible, give a small test dose (e.g., haloperidol 5 mg) and wait 1 hour to see if it is tolerated.

  2. Then begin haloperidol 10–15 mg/day, chlorpromazine 300–400 mg/day, or the equivalent. Use tid or qd schedule initially, then switch to bid or qid after 1–2 weeks. A qd schedule is usually well tolerated and helps insomnia. It may be necessary to increase to 500 mg/day of chlorpromazine, 15–20 mg/day of haloperidol, or the equivalent. Rarely go higher. If side effects become a problem, begin antiparkinsonism drugs and/or reduce the dosage and increase more slowly.

  3. If the patient is wild and needs immediate control, and effective physical control is not readily available, consider more rapid tranquilization, e.g., haloperidol 5 mg IM every hour 3 or 4 times (or, perhaps more effective, haloperidol 5 mg + lorazepam 2–4 mg IM in the same syringe). [Droperidol, 5 mg IM, may be the most effective acute tranquilizer but is not approved by the FDA for that purpose (but it *is* used).] Monitor carefully for hypotension or oversedation. Once the patient is under control, switch to the preceding daily schedule.

- Disease control is *cognitive as well as behavioral:* The goal is not just to "quiet" the patient. Improvement is slow and often partial. Increasing socialization is an early sign of a drug response. Agitated disruptive behavior usually improves in the first several days. The thought disorder disappears over weeks or months. Traditional antipsychotics improve the *positive symptoms* of psychosis (e.g., hallucinations, delusions, bizarre behavior), but unfortunately they usually do not change the *negative symptoms* (e.g., flat affect, social impairment)—a major problem (addition of low-dose SSRI occasionally helps). Patients who are "acutely crazy" are *most* likely to respond well, as are those with good premorbid functioning who are having their first psychotic episode. If there are significant obsessive-compulsive symptoms, consider a trial of clomipramine. If a depression appears, consider switching to an atypical antipsychotic: Antidepressants are of modest help at best.

- If a patient *does not respond*: Switch to another drug of a different type. However, the unimproved patient needs at least one 2–3 week trial at a higher dose of an antipsychotic before you conclude that he or she does not respond to medication. There is rarely any reason to use two different antipsychotics simultaneously. The most common cause for lack of response is underdosage (and noncompliance), but always be wary that the patient may have an organic psychosis.

- *Once improvement has occurred:* Maintain drug levels over 1–2 months and then consider reducing to maintenance levels. If this is the first episode of an acute psychosis in a previously well-functioning patient, consider discontinuing the medication in 6–12 months. If this episode is one of many, the patient may need maintenance medication for years.

- *Antipsychotic maintenance therapy:* Decrease dosage slowly (over weeks to months) to one third or one quarter of the acute dose. If a relapse begins, increase the dose. About 90% of patients relapse (during first 24 months) without medication, and 40% or more relapse while taking them. Teach the patient to recognize her own developing relapse so it can be caught early.

Traditional antipsychotics are often unpleasant to take, so compliance is a major problem with outpatients (particularly those patients who are suspicious and paranoid). Pay attention to and work vigorously to control side effects (particularly akathisia). If the patient is reluctant to take daily medication, consider the long-acting depot forms of two very potent antipsychotics: fluphenazine decanoate and haloperidol decanoate. They can be given IM every 2–4 weeks in very low doses (e.g., fluphenazine decanoate, 12.5–25 mg IM every 2 weeks, or haloperidol decanoate, 50–100 or more mg IM every month). The relapse rate may be slightly increased at these doses, but side effects and compliance usually are improved. (In fact, depot medication may be preferable, whether or not the patient is noncompliant, particularly in the medication-refractory patient.)

Atypical Antipsychotics

There are currently four new antipsychotics available in the United States, with a fifth likely to be available by the turn of the century. Four of the five quickly have become the initial **treatment of choice** for schizophrenia and other psychotic conditions (3). Choose one of them first because

1. They have many fewer side effects than the traditional antipsychotics. Thus, compliance is likely to be much improved.
2. They are at least equally effective in treating the positive symptoms of schizophrenia (4), and all (?) seem to be effective at treating the **negative symptoms** as well.
3. They may produce less cognitive impairment than the traditional medications.
4. They seem to allow the patient a higher quality of life than the traditional antipsychotics (5).
5. With the exception of clozapine, they appear quite safe.
6. Early studies have found them to have a comparatively low relapse rate (6).

Although these medications seem to be a marked improvement over earlier antipsychotics, research sufficient to confirm their superiority unambiguously has not yet been done. However, it does appear as though they all work through some variation of the same mechanism: They all have a modest to moderate effect at blocking the D_2 receptor and, unlike the older drugs, a moderate ability to block the 5-HT_{2A} receptor. Why that psychobiologic pattern should make them superior antipsychotics is unknown at this time.

Clozapine, the only one of the five medications that is not a first-line drug (due to an uncommon but very dangerous side effect of agranulocytosis), has been shown fairly clearly to be the drug of choice for treatment-resistant schizophrenia. There is suggestive, but less complete and convincing, evidence that one or more of the other newer medications also are effective in patients in which the older antipsychotics have failed (7). Too few comparison studies among these medications have been done to allow the clinician to decide which one is preferable for which patient. They all seem to be roughly equivalent. They currently also are being used fairly widely (and successfully) in conditions like bipolar disorder (mania), intermittent explosive disorder, and in geriatric patients with agitated behavior and/or dementia. The limits of their utility have not yet been reached. One negative feature (at this time) to these medications is that they all are quite expensive. Also, they may, as a group, require 2–3 weeks before significant improvement is seen.

Finally, most general principles followed when treating patients with the older medications also apply here: e.g., (a) a complete trial takes about 8 weeks, (b) a patient who smokes heavily generally requires a higher dose of medication due to increased clearance, and (c) if a patient is prone to relapse when taken off medication, any one of these drugs appears to be an appropriate choice for a maintenance regimen. There are two situations in which the traditional antipsychotics still are required. First, because only ziprasidone (not yet released in the U.S.) has an injectable form, acute psychosis frequently requires the use of a traditional antipsychotic like IM haloperidol. (Research studies suggest that both risperidone and olanzapine will shortly be available in an injectable form also.) Second, none of the new antipsychotics are available in a depot form either, so the noncompliant or irresponsible patient may require a traditional depot medication.

Specific New Medications

- **Clozapine** (Clozaril), a new and different antipsychotic, should be used with schizophrenic patients who cannot tolerate or are refractory to traditional medications. Marked improvement occurs in almost 30% of treatment-resistant chronic patients; modest improvement in another 10%–20%. Unlike other antipsychotics, clozapine may improve symptoms of apathy, withdrawal, anhedonia, and flat affect—a "significant cure" in a few patients.

  After a thorough medical (laboratory) examination, begin dosage at 25 mg and increase to 300–400 daily (bid-tid schedule) over 2–3 weeks. (It is very expensive—the median daily dosage of 400 mg costs $4,000 or more per year.) A response may take weeks or even months. Upper limit is 900 mg/day but be very cautious above 600 mg because some side effects are related to dose and speed of increase, e.g., *sedation,* grand mal *seizures* (unusual under 300 mg; 5% of patients over 600 mg; do not use in patients with a history of a seizure disorder). Other side effects include sialorrhea, *weight gain,* tachycardia, hypotension, fever, and elevated liver enzymes.

The life-threatening side effect is **agranulocytosis:** about 1% of patients; usually during months 1–6 (but possible anytime); requires *weekly* WBCs with diff for approximately 2 years, then every 2 weeks (stop medication if the WBC < 3,000 or granulocytes < 1,500); apparently not dose-related. If WBCs drop below 2,000, never rechallenge the patient with clozapine. Do not use in patients with known blood dyscrasias or who are taking drugs with similar effects on the WBCs (e.g., carbamazepine). TAKE THESE GUIDELINES SERIOUSLY.

- **Risperidone** (Risperdal) was the second new antipsychotic released in the U.S. It has fewer side effects than previous antipsychotics, is safe in overdose, and seems to affect both positive and negative symptoms. Begin with 0.5–1 mg bid; the ideal final dose for most patients is 4–6 mg/day (can take as a single dose). It is usually effective and well tolerated at that level, although the risk for EPS increases significantly above 6 mg/day (8). TD has been seen with this medication; weight gain is minor.

- **Olanzapine** (Zyprexa) is effective when taken in a once-daily dose of 10–25 mg (begin with 5 mg/day). It seems to produce less EPS than risperidone but produces considerably more *weight gain* as well as sedation and postural hypotension. In most regards, other than side effects, it seems equivalent to risperidone.

- **Quetiapine** (Seroquel) may be slightly less effective than the other new antipsychotics, although that impression may reflect an insufficiency of well-done studies rather than reality. Its side effects are similar to those of olanzapine, although perhaps not as severe, but *weight gain* and orthostatic hypotension may be problems. The range of dosage is unusually broad, with clinically similar patients requiring anywhere from 100–750 mg daily (bid recommended).

- **Ziprasidone** (Zeldox) has not been released in the U.S. as of mid-1999 but seems certain to receive FDA approval by the beginning of 2000. It seems to be a very effective medication that has the advantage of very minimal weight gain (if any at all). Its side effects tend to be GI complaints: nausea, abdominal pain, dyspepsia, and constipation, although they are generally mild. Ziprasidone also has the advantage of being available in pill, liquid, and IM form. Finally, it acts as a 5-HT$_{1A}$

agonist and thus may be an effective antianxiety agent as well. It looks promising; time will tell.

MOOD STABILIZERS

Lithium Carbonate

- Li$^+$; atomic #3
- Slow-release form, Eskalith CR, Lithobid Slow-Release Tablets

Indications for Use

Recommended for:

1. **"Classic" acute bipolar disorder, manic** (9): Lithium is the drug of choice for stabilization of an acute manic attack (80% of patients normalize), although due to the usual 7–10 day delay in clinical onset, an additional drug *may* be needed initially for control. Best for "classic" bipolar disorder; for "rapid-cyclers" use anticonvulsants instead (only about 1/3 respond to Li).
2. **Acute depression:** *bipolar* (good; up to 80% respond but slow to act, takes 3–6 weeks) and *unipolar* (about 1/3 respond; thus a second-choice drug). Definitely consider the addition of Li to augment a partial response to another (any other) antidepressant—50% respond (usually quickly; slightly more than 1 week).
3. **Long-term prophylaxis of mania in a bipolar patient:** It is quite effective at preventing recurrences when coupled with an anticonvulsant. Be careful of chronic renal toxicity.

Other possible uses:

- Prophylaxis for bipolar disorder, depressed and for major depression.
- May assist (usually) or replace antipsychotics in treatment of a few patients with schizoaffective disorder.
- May help control mood swings, *impulsive aggression,* and *explosive outbursts* regardless of cause. Also, retarded patients with aggressiveness and/or self-mutilation.
- Curiously, it is effective in chronic prophylactic treatment of *cluster headaches.*

Mechanisms of Action

The reasons for the clinical effects are poorly understood, although Li does enhance presynaptic serotonergic neurotransmission, seems to reduce pre- and postsynaptic dopamine transmission, and increases plasma NE levels.

Pharmacokinetics

Lithium is quickly absorbed from the GI tract (completely absorbed in 8 hours) and develops a peak plasma level in 1–3 hours. It is *not* protein bound or metabolized and is excreted by the kidney. The CSF concentration is 30%–60% of that in plasma and equivalent to that in RBCs. It is concentrated by bone and by thyroid (4–5 times that in plasma).

Lithium can *only* be used safely if blood concentrations are monitored carefully (oral dosage is *not* an adequate measure). To obtain consistent levels, draw blood 12 hours after the last dose (e.g., take evening dose and then draw before breakfast). The lithium half-life is 18–36 hours (fastest in youth, slowest in elderly); a constant oral dosage requires 5–8 days to reach steady state. Once a steady state is reached, the lithium level is proportional to the daily oral dose (and determined by the renal clearance).

Side Effects

The number and severity of side effects increase with elevated or rapidly changing/increasing Li blood levels. A slight change in blood level (0.1–0.2 mEq/L) may alter dramatically the number or intensity of the side effects. Minor side effects (tremor, impaired coordination, dysarthria, thirst, anorexia, and GI distress) commonly occur at therapeutic levels (0.8–1.5 mEq/L), and serious effects (nausea and vomiting, slurred speech, diarrhea, coarse tremors, severe ataxia, confusion, delirium, seizures, coma, death) may occur at only slightly higher levels (e.g., as low as 2.0–2.5 mEq/L but more commonly at 3–5 mEq/L). Some evidence suggests that mild side effects can be controlled with a daily dietary supplement of 20–40 mEq of K^+. Lithium has a very narrow margin of safety and is a dangerous drug in overdosage. It should be given cautiously (or not given at all) in patients who are dehydrated, febrile, have sodium depletion (kidney reabsorbs more lithium), or have major renal or cardiovascular disease. Brain-damaged patients and the elderly are at risk for side effects even at low blood levels, so use with care.

Normal subjects administered lithium report irritability and emotional lability, anxiety, mild depression, tiredness and malaise, weakness, inability to concentrate, impaired memory, and slowed reaction time. Patients taking lithium often experience a "lithium-induced dysphoria," and 25%–50% stop lithium AMA. Unlike other psychoactive medication, sedation is *not* a side effect.

Specific side effects include the following:

- **Neurologic:**

  EEG—Usually shows increased amplitude and generalized slowing (in 50% of patients at therapeutic blood levels).

  Headaches, occasional slurred speech.

  Toxicity:

    Confusion, poor concentration, and clouding of consciousness, leading to delirium, coma, and death.

    Cerebellar effects—dysarthria, ataxia, nystagmus, severe incoordination.

  Basal ganglia effects—Parkinsonian symptoms, choreiform movements.

  Seizures—grand mal; status epilepticus.

- **Neuromuscular:**

  Hand tremor (fine, fast) that does not respond to anticholinergics. Occurs in 50% of the patients started on lithium but the incidence decreases with time (5% of long-term patients). Treat with β-blockers (e.g., propranolol orally 30–80 mg/day).

  Muscular weakness—one third of patients during the first week of treatment; transient.

  Neuromuscular toxicity—hyperactive reflexes, fasciculations, paralysis.

- **Kidney:**

  Polyuria and polydipsia—secondary to a vasopressin-resistant diabetes insipidus-like syndrome. Reversible and occurs in 50% of all new patients (5% of all chronics).

  Reversible oliguric renal failure with acute lithium intoxication.

Possible irreversible nephrotoxic effect in a few chronic
patients—focal interstitial cortical fibrosis with tubular atrophy and sclerotic glomeruli. Look for a gradually increasing blood lithium in patients taking a constant oral dose. There is increased serum creatinine
and an increased 24-hour urine volume. Poorly characterized currently, this serious effect of chronic
lithium administration may limit the ability to use
lithium prophylactically in some.

- **Blood:**

  Leukocytosis (10,000–14,000 WBCs; neutrophilia with lym-
  phocytopenia)—Common and reversible, it is persistent but periodic while the patient is taking lithium.

  Occasional increased ESR.

- **GI:**

  30% of patients have GI symptoms in the early weeks of
  treatment—gastric irritation, nausea, anorexia, diarrhea, bloating, abdominal pain (a switch to lithium
  citrate may relieve symptoms).

- **Heart:**

  T-wave flattening or inversion (common but reversible).

  Unusual—myocarditis, SA block, primary AV block; ventricular irritability and perhaps sudden death (particularly in older males with cardiac pathology; more common at toxic levels).

- **Thyroid:**

  Lithium may produce hypothyroidism with (10% of
  chronic patients) or without a goiter. Measure TSH.
  Low-dose thyroxine may help but consult an endocri-
  nologist.

- **Other:**

  Impaired memory.

  Lithium accumulates in bone—no known harmful effects.

  Occasional maculopapular rash, acne, and also (rarely)
  alopecia, ulceration, and exacerbation of psoriasis.

  Weight gain in 10% or more of patients. Partly related to a
  Li-induced reactive hypoglycemia.

  Occasional benign reversible exophthalmos.

  Hyperparathyroidism—increased serum calcium and para-
  thyroid hormone, usually without other symptoms.

Most side effects disappear with chronic lithium administration. The side effects which tend to be include tremor, polyuria, leukocytosis, goiter, and elevated blood sugar.

In Pregnancy:

1. Lithium crosses the placenta freely and can produce cardiac malformations (Ebstein's anomaly and others), although they seem to be infrequent. Pregnant women should avoid lithium unless the risks of a "manic pregnancy" outweigh the small risk of fetal malformations. Such infants are also at risk for nephrogenic diabetes insipidus, hypoglycemia, and euthyroid goiter.

2. Lithium in milk is 30%–100% of the maternal blood level; thus, these mothers should not breast-feed.

3. Lithium clearance increases 50%–100% early in pregnancy and returns to normal at delivery; thus, a dosage raised during pregnancy must be immediately reduced or the mother will become toxic.

Drug Interactions

- Diuretics—Thiazides decrease lithium clearance and increase blood levels; furosemide, ethacrynic acid, spironolactone, and triamterene may also. Mannitol, urea, and acetazolamide decrease blood levels. Tetracyclines, indomethacin, phenylbutazone, and methyldopa may increase lithium blood levels.

- Haloperidol (and other high potency neuroleptics)—a (usually) reversible neurotoxicity may occur in some patients at higher doses of antipsychotic (confusion, disorientation, etc.). Potentially life-threatening—watch for it.

- Chlorpromazine may increase the rate of lithium excretion.

- Tricyclic antidepressants may act *synergistically* with lithium.

- Aminophylline increases lithium excretion.

- Lithium probably prolongs the neuromuscular blocking effect of succinylcholine.

Treatment Principles

- *Select appropriate patients.* Screen for serious medical illness. Preadministration laboratory evaluation should include
  - CBC, BUN, UA;
  - Serum creatinine;

- T_3, T_4, thyroid examination;
- Serum Na^+ if there is reason to question the patient's electrolyte status;
- ECG if the physical or history suggests cardiac disease;
- If chronic use of lithium is expected, obtain 24-hour urine volume, creatinine clearance, and protein excretion.

- *Treatment of acute mania:* The goal is to produce a therapeutic blood level (1.2–1.4 mEq/L) and maintain it until a clinical effect is seen (usually 7–10 days after an appropriate level is attained). Begin lithium 300 mg PO bid-tid. Always give in divided doses (usually tid-qid; bid-tid with slow-release form). Increase by 300 mg every 2–3 days (typical effective oral dose is 1,200–2,400 mg/day). Slow-release total oral dosage should be the same as that of regular Li.

  Methods to determine the appropriate steady-state dose of Li based on blood levels after a single initial test dose of Li have been developed. As yet, none can be considered standard, but some appear promising and would help speed up the treatment of manic patients.

  Because acute mania is not controlled by lithium for 2–3 weeks, it may be necessary on the first day of treatment to begin a benzodiazepine (e.g., lorazepam, 2–4 mg PO/IM q2 hours every 2 hours with an average of 20 or more mg/day initially) or an antipsychotic (e.g., haloperidol 5–20 mg/day, in divided doses) if the patient is excessively agitated. Both provide rapid control of the psychomotor activity while the lithium acts more gradually but is more specific for control of the affect and ideation of mania.

  Once the mania begins to remit, the *blood Li level may increase* (mechanism?)—keep watch. Maintain a therapeutic level until the mania is completely controlled (measure blood levels every 1–2 weeks). Lithium is best for "classic" long-period bipolar disorder; if response is poor, consider adding an anticonvulsant (e.g., valproic acid).

Maintenance

- *Treatment of mania:* If a patient has a history of recurrent mania, continue lithium after the acute attack (drug of choice). An effective maintenance blood level is 0.8 mEq/L (range, 0.6–1.0). When stable, measure the blood level every

2–3 months (be aware that a crash diet or strenuous exercise program may change the patient's level). Unfortunately, non-compliance is common, so work with the patient. If you choose to discontinue the Li, taper *slowly* (10).

Teach the patient to be alert to side effects that suggest toxicity and measure lithium level if they occur. Lithium level increases with sodium loss so advise the patient to be aware of changes in dietary salt intake, sweating, and hot climates (although Li *may* be lost more rapidly than sodium, causing the Li level to fall).

Concern about gradual lithium-induced renal toxicity is decreasing: standard measures of serum creatinine, UA, BUN, protein excretion, and 24-hour urine volume every 6–12 months may not be necessary (11). Monitor thyroid function—T_3, T_4, and physical examination every 6 months.

- Lithium prophylaxis of mania/depression is only partial. If a patient on maintenance lithium shows signs of developing mania, raise the lithium to an acute therapeutic level (50% or more respond). If the patient develops a severe depression, begin an antidepressant (although a few patients will have developed subclinical hypothyroidism 2° to Li, so consider thyroid supplementation instead). However, equally effective medication for prophylaxis may include carbamazepine, valproate, other anticonvulsants, and clonazepam; Li and valproate may be the maintenance combination of choice in difficult patients.

Other Mood Stabilizers

There has been a blossoming of the use of selected anticonvulsants as mood stabilizers (12). Carbamazepine, and then valproic acid, have been used for years for most of the same indications as lithium. In fact, because of equal or superior efficacy and greater safety, particularly with valproic acid, these drugs have gradually been replacing Li as the first-line medication. More recently, several additional anticonvulsants have been added to their number: lamotrigine, gabapentin, and topiramate. Moreover, combinations of Li and one of the various mood stabilizers or combinations of different mood stabilizers seem to be particularly effective (13).

- **Carbamazepine** (Tegretol) is an anticonvulsant that seems to be as effective as lithium for treating acute mania (better than lithium for *rapid cyclers*) and bipolar depression, and for mania prophylaxis. Moreover, it may be of use in treating certain violent individuals. Doses are typically 800 mg/day or more (blood level = 6–8 mg/L). Begin slowly, raise over 2–3 weeks, and check blood level 5–6 times during the first month because the drug induces its own metabolism. Side effects include fatigue, nausea, ataxia, and diplopia. Allergic rashes are common (5%–15%), as are dose-related side effects like *sedation* and dizziness. Initial, mild, benign leukopenia is common (10%), but watch for more serious problems of aplastic anemia, *agranulocytosis,* and hepatic toxicity that develops over months or years. Get a CBC and diff at least with every drug blood level.
- **Valproic acid** (Depakene) has a similar spectrum of utility (rapid cycling bipolars, particularly mania and mania prophylaxis but also depression) but with a different and safer side-effect spectrum (*sedation,* tremor, rare hepatotoxicity) (14). Half-life is 12 or more hours: maintain a blood level modestly above 50 ng/mL (start at 250 mg bid, but may require 1,000 or more mg/day). In most situations, valproic acid is a better choice than carbamazepine.

Too little is known about the three other anticonvulsants currently approved to treat bipolar disorder, **lamotrigine** (15) (Lamictal), **gabapentin** (16) (Neurontin), and **topiramate** (Topamaz), to distinguish one from another or to know whether any is superior to either of the two medications above. Time and experience should allow us to rank order these five medications.

Finally, there is increasing evidence that several of the new antipsychotic medications may, by themselves, be useful drugs for treating bipolar I disorder, e.g., clozapine (17), risperidone (18), and olanzapine (19).

ANTIDEPRESSANT DRUGS

Three groups of antidepressant drugs are in common use: tricyclic antidepressants (TCAs), newer antidepressants, and monoamine oxidase inhibitors (MAOIs) (Table 23.4). Combinations of these drugs are also occasionally helpful. Until recently the TCAs have been the first choice in treating depressions, but the newer antidepressants (the SSRIs and others) have shown themselves to be just as effective as the TCAs in treating dysthymia, major depression, and a number of other disorders as well as having fewer side effects. Thus, these newer medications have supplanted the TCAs as the initial therapeutic choice for most situations (except for cost). Lithium carbonate can improve some major depressions, and the antipsychotic drugs are essential in psychotic depression. The MAOIs are effective but generally are used only after 2 or 3 other medications have failed.

TABLE 23.4   Antidepressant Drugs in Common Use

Drugs available (in U.S.)	Anticholinergic	Sedation	Dose (mg/day)
TCAs			
imipramine (Tofranil)	4 +	3 +	75–300
amitriptyline (Elavil, Endep)	5 +	5 +	75–300
clomipramine (Anafranil)	4 +	3 +	75–250
doxepin (Sinequan, Adapin)	4 +	5 +	75–300
desipramine (Norpramin)	1 +	1 +	75–300
nortriptyline (Pamelor)	3 +	2 +	40–150
protriptyline (Vivactil)	3 +	1 +	20–60
trimipramine (Surmontil)	3 +	4 +	75–200
Newer antidepressants			
alprazolam (Xanax)	1 +	5 +	2–6
amoxapine (Asendin)	2 +	3 +	200–300
buproprion (Wellbutrin)	0–1 +	0–1 +	200–450
maprotiline (Ludiomil)	2 +	2 +	50–225
mirtazapine (Remeron)	2 +	3 +	30–45
trazodone (Desyrel)	1 +	3 +	100–600
venlafaxine (Effexor)	1 +	1 +	75–375
citalopram (Celexa)	0–1 +	1 +	30–60
fluoxetine (Prozac)	0–1 +	0–1 +	10–40 +
fluvoxamine (Luvox)	0–1 +	0–1 +	100–300
nefazodone (Serzone)	0–1 +	2 +	300–600
paroxetine (Paxil)	0–1 +	0–1 +	20–50
sertraline (Zoloft)	0–1 +	0–1 +	50–200
MAOIs			
phenelzine (Nardil)	1 +	1 +	30–90
isocarboxazid (Marplan)	1 +	1 +	10–30
tranylcypromine (Parnate)	1 +	0	20–60

Tricyclic Antidepressants (TCAs)

Indications for Use

Recommended for:

1. Major depression—Particularly with vegetative symptoms and a diurnal variation (70%–75% of patients respond).
2. Bipolar disorder, depressed or mixed—Particularly if there are vegetative symptoms. Lithium may be useful as well.
3. Short-term maintenance therapy in patients with resolved major depression or bipolar disease.
4. Prophylaxis in patients with severe recurrent major depression.
5. Psychotic depression (hallucinations, delusions, paranoia, etc.)—Must be combined with antipsychotics (although ECT may be preferable for some).
6. Postpartum depressions that are severe.

Other uses:

- Dysthymic disorder—Mild chronic depressions which haven't responded to newer antidepressants deserve a trial of TCAs.
- Atypical depression—Patients with significant anxiety, hypochondriasis, and neurotic complaints, as an alternative to MAOIs.
- Panic disorder, with or without agoraphobia—one among several choices.
- OCD—Particularly those patients who also have a depressed mood. Clomipramine is uniquely effective with OCD.
- PTSD—One among several choices.
- Selected patients with chronic pain (with or without depression).
- Childhood conditions—Both enuresis and school phobia may respond to low doses of a TCA.

TCAs should *not* be used routinely in the various minor depressive syndromes.

Mechanisms of Action

The effects of TCAs on CNS neurotransmitters are complex and vary from one tricyclic to another. Therapeutic impact is *thought* to be related to some combination of CNS interneuronal NE increase due to presynaptic NE reuptake blockade and to the sensitization of postsynaptic neurons to serotonin. Although affecting both systems, *secondary amines* (desipramine, protriptyline, and nortriptyline) may preferentially raise NE levels, whereas *tertiary amines* (amitriptyline, imipramine, and doxepin) have a greater effect on serotonin, a fact used to account for some interpatient response differences. In summary, however, knowledge is incomplete and we use these drugs based on "clinical wisdom."

Pharmacokinetics

TCAs are absorbed rapidly and completely from the GI tract, undergo an enterohepatic cycle, and develop peak plasma levels in 2–8 hours. TCAs are highly bound to plasma and tissue proteins and are fat soluble; free TCA is only about 1% of the total body load. They are metabolized by the liver and excreted by the kidney. The half-life ranges from several hours to more than 2 days.

Well-studied plasma blood levels are available for imipramine, nortriptyline, desipramine, and amitriptyline. Do not measure them routinely. Indications include

1. Treatment failure—Interindividual plasma levels vary markedly after the same oral dose (up to 30-fold differences), so always consider an ineffective plasma level when explaining a treatment failure. Therapeutic range is 150–300 ng/mL for imipramine (+ its metabolite, desipramine), amitriptyline (+ nortriptyline), or desipramine, and 50–160 ng/mL for nortriptyline.
2. Therapeutic window—Some TCAs may have a *therapeutic window* (e.g., nortriptyline and possibly desipramine). The drugs are less effective outside this range, whereas others seem to have no therapeutic upper limit (e.g., imipramine—range is limited only by side effects).
3. Suspected patient noncompliance.
4. Patients with significant side effects on a usual oral dose; they may have an excessively high plasma level.
5. Patients with cardiac disease—attempt to maintain a low (but effective) plasma level.
6. The medically unstable patient (particularly the elderly).
7. Overdose—plasma levels are mandatory.

Side Effects

Side effects are frequent and usually mild but can be serious or fatal (particularly cardiac effects in TCA overdoses) and are more common in the elderly.

- Anticholinergic:
    Dry mouth
    Blurred vision (near vision)
    Constipation, urinary hesitancy
- Autonomic:
    Sweating
    Impotence, ejaculatory dysfunction
- Cardiac:
In normal dosages: tachycardia and ECG changes (T-wave flattening, increased PR and QT interval)
In overdose: PVCs, ventricular arrhythmias, AV block and BBB, CHF and cardiac arrest
- Other:
    Orthostatic hypotension (can be severe)
    Sedation
    Restlessness, insomnia
    Rashes, allergic reactions
    Weight gain (a common cause of patient noncompliance)
    Anorexia, nausea and vomiting
    EEG changes
    Tremor (fine, rapid, usually hands and fingers)
    Confusion (in elderly)
    Seizures in patients who are predisposed

Tolerance usually develops to the anticholinergic and sedative side effects. Use cautiously in the elderly and in patients with BPH; avoid in patients with narrow-angle glaucoma. Pregnancy is not an absolute contraindication for TCA use, although there is suggestive (but not convincing) evidence of teratogenicity; avoid use in the first trimester if possible. Severe hypotension occasionally can limit drug use (it is least with nortriptyline and doxepin).

Most worrisome are the cardiac effects. There have been a few reports of sudden death from presumed arrhythmias. Patients with preexisting heart disease (particularly bundle-branch disease) and/or hypertension (e.g., the elderly) are at risk for any of the cardiac side effects. Do *not* use after an acute MI or while in CHF. The danger is greatest with higher doses (e.g., after an overdose with a TCA).

There are wide differences between agents in their ability to produce some side effects, and these should be considered when choosing a drug. The presence of side effects is *not* a good indication that a therapeutic plasma level has been reached.

Certain psychiatric conditions may be adversely affected by TCAs. (a) Schizophrenia may be made worse. (b) A depressed bipolar patient may become manic (10% or more; "may" be lower with other antidepressants).

A withdrawal syndrome occurs in some patients who have been taking high doses of TCAs (e.g., imipramine 150–300 mg/day) for weeks or months. If medication is stopped abruptly, symptoms begin in 1–2 days and include anxiety, headache, myalgia, chills, malaise, and nausea. Withdraw the medication gradually (e.g., 25–50 mg/wk).

Drug Interactions
- TCA plasma level is increased (at times dangerously) by methylphenidate, Antabuse, MAOIs, antipsychotics, SSRIs, exogenous thyroid, cimetidine, and guanethidine.
- TCA plasma level is decreased (*frequently* below therapeutic range) by barbiturates, alcohol, carbamazepine, phenytoin, doxycycline, and *smoking* (may need to monitor level in heavy smokers).
- CNS depression occurs with antipsychotics, anticonvulsants, hypnotic-sedatives, and alcohol.
- TCAs impair the antihypertensive effect of methyldopa, guanethidine, and bethanidine.
- There is a synergistic anticholinergic effect with other central anticholinergics—may produce a toxic psychosis.
- Marked hypertension can be caused by administration of TCAs with sympathomimetic drugs (e.g., isoproterenol, epinephrine, phenylephrine, amphetamines).
- TCAs may dangerously increase the half-life of anticoagulants (e.g., Dicumarol)—monitor prothrombin time.

Treatment Principles
- Identify the patient likely to benefit from a TCA (remember: for many patients the starting drug of choice may be one of the newer antidepressants).
  1. Appropriate clinical presentation.
  2. Past personal history of good TCA response.
  3. Past family history of good TCA response.

- Unless side effects are likely to be a problem, begin with a tertiary TCA. They are metabolized in the liver to 2° TCAs (imipramine to desipramine; amitriptyline to nortriptyline) and thus both the 3° and 2° TCAs are present in the body.
- Side effects may be useful (e.g., consider amitriptyline or doxepin in the agitated depressive, desipramine in the elderly with anticholinergic intolerance, protriptyline if sedation is a problem, and nortriptyline if hypotension is excessive).
- One technique for treating depression with TCAs is:

  Begin imipramine 50 mg PO HS (or equivalent—less in elderly; more in the obese) and increase by 25–50 mg every 2–3 days until 150 mg is reached. If side effects interfere, slow down.

  Hold dosage at 150 mg for 1 week. If depression remains, increase to 200 mg (50 mg during the day, 150 at HS).

  Hold dosage at 200 mg for 1 week and then increase in 50-mg steps to 300 mg (150 mg in divided doses during the day, 150 mg at HS). Consider hospitalizing the patient for trials above 200 mg/day. Maintain at 300 mg for 2 to 3 weeks. It is important to do complete trials, if side effect problems allow. If depression remains,

    1. Has patient been taking medication?
    2. Has a therapeutic window been passed?
    3. Measure plasma level.

  If the patient is unimproved, consider

    1. A newer antidepressant or a different TCA.
    2. ECT.
    3. An MAOI. Allow 1–2 weeks for transfer.
    4. After 2–3 unsuccessful trials, reevaluate the diagnosis.

  With a good response, sleep and appetite usually return first, then an improved mood. There is usually a 1-to 3-week delay in the therapeutic effect, so do not stop medication prematurely.

- Never give a worrisomely depressed or seriously suicidal patient a prescription for more than 1,000 mg of imipramine (or equivalent).
- If treating a psychotic depression, use a TCA and an antipsychotic simultaneously.

- If treating a depression in a bipolar patient taking lithium, continue the lithium if it has been effective prophylactically. The lithium *may* help prevent a manic overshoot.
- If treating a phobic-anxiety disorder, expect improvement with a lower dosage (e.g., 100 mg).
- Simultaneous use of a TCA and an MAOI is currently discouraged by the FDA but is often useful.
- Maintenance care: In a successfully treated patient, maintain the medication at acute levels for 6 months. If the patient has had a recurrence of a major depression, consider long-term TCA maintenance at full dosage (reduces likelihood of a relapse by 50%). Consider lithium maintenance in a recurrent bipolar illness. If there is no previous history of illness, gradually withdraw the medication. Recognize as many as one fourth of the improved patients relapse during the first 4 months and a significant number of patients (30% or more) maintain a chronic low-level depression, even though treated successfully for the acute illness ("double depression"). Depression, all too often, is a chronic illness.
- Clomipramine (Anafranil) is a little special: Approved for OCD but an effective TCA antidepressant with a significant serotonin effect. Range of effectiveness is closer to some of the new antidepressants (although it has all the TCA side effects).
- TCA overdose is life-threatening and should be treated on a medical inpatient unit. Dangerously high plasma levels may continue for more than 1 week.
- Although generally not considered drugs of abuse, illicit use of amitriptyline to produce anticholinergic intoxication has been reported. Watch for it.

Newer Antidepressants

The following medications have become the *drugs of first choice,* to be used before TCAs and MAOIs in most cases. The primary reason for using "newer antidepressants" is their different side-effect spectrums and toxicity: They differ little from TCAs in effectiveness, disorders treated, or speed of onset. Their mechanisms of action are diverse. Curiously, both sertraline (20) and fluvoxamine (21) alone have been found effective in psychotic depressions. The key drugs include:

- **alprazolam** (Xanax): A benzodiazepine that *may* be antidepressant at higher doses; few side effects except sedation and risk of *addiction*; safe in overdose. (A "second-string" antidepressant.)
- **amoxapine** (Asendin): A metabolite of the antipsychotic loxapine; side effects similar to TCAs; *may* be of particular use in psychotic depressions. Be careful of overdoses.
- **bupropion** (Wellbutrin): An effective drug with few side effects and safe in overdose; can produce insomnia and sweating; may be more likely to produce seizures, so go slow and avoid patients at risk. Probably one of the better new drugs. It is often the choice for patients who experience anorgasmia from the SSRIs. Aim for 300–400 mg/day in *divided doses* (also available in slow-release form: Wellbutrin SR).
- **maprotiline** (Ludiomil): Like TCAs; less cardiotoxicity in overdose.
- **mirtazapine** (Remeron): An α_2-adrenergic antagonist, so a peculiar mechanism of action. Weight gain and sedation are problems. Perhaps an anxiolytic. *No* drug interactions.
- **nefazodone** (Serzone): Similar to trazodone but without the sexual dysfunction. Cardiotoxicity not a problem and very little anticholinergic and histaminergic activity. Side effects include sedation, dizziness, and headache. Do not use with MAOIs.
- **reboxetine:** Not available in the U.S. although likely to be released soon (22). Shows significant promise. Limited side effects [particularly nausea and also sexual anorgasmia and impotence (in one-third)] and a unique mechanism of action: a "pure NE blocker."
- **SEROTONIN REUPTAKE BLOCKERS (SSRIs):** As a group these antidepressants are safe and effective. They have similar (modest) side effects [particularly nausea and also sexual anorgasmia and impotence (in one-third)] but if one medication cannot be tolerated, another one might be fine.

    Fluoxetine (Prozac)—Little sedation or anticholinergic effects (perhaps daytime sedation in a few); does produce GI upset, rashes, sexual inhibition, insomnia, and restlessness. Clearly effective in mild-to-moderate depressions and may be the medication to start with rather than a TCA. Try 20 mg daily [one dose—long half-life (days)], although some patients require 40 mg whereas a few are okay with 20 mg every other day. *May* not be as effective as TCAs at preventing relapse.

Sertraline (Zoloft) is similar to fluoxetine; safe and mild side effects—nausea, diarrhea, tremor, insomnia, somnolence, dry mouth, ejaculatory delay; one dose/day of 50–200 mg. **Paroxetine** (Paxil) is also similar; daily dose is 20–50 mg. **Fluvoxamine** (Luvox) is an SSRI similar to the others, although it is FDA approved for OCD, not for depression (however, it is used "off label" for depression). **Citalopram** (Celexa) is an *almost pure* SSRI blocker (slightly less expensive than similar medications; no known drug–drug interactions).

Three drug–drug combinations are of concern. (a) Fluoxetine + an MAOI produces a dangerous *serotonin syndrome* (23): restlessness, tremor and myoclonus, hyperreflexia, diarrhea, and diaphoresis, leading possibly to confusion and death. Wait 5 weeks to begin an MAOI after stopping fluoxetine; wait 2–3 weeks going from an MAOI to fluoxetine. (b) Fluoxetine raises (sometimes dramatically) blood levels of TCAs, trazodone, maprotiline, carbamazepine, the benzodiazepines, and (probably) others, so be careful. (c) L-tryptophan + fluoxetine can produce myoclonic jerks. Finally, early concern was expressed by a few about the possibility that fluoxetine (and other SSRIs) may produce (or worsen) suicidal and/or aggressive impulses; appears to be a "red herring" (but).

Trazodone (Desyrel): Free of anticholinergic and most cardiac effects; produces orthostatic hypotension, sedation (useful if insomnia is a major problem), GI distress, headaches, and (rarely) *priapism.* Start low (e.g., 50 mg) and raise to the 200–300 mg range. Is it less effective than others? It is frequently used as a safe hypnotic.

Venlafaxine (Effexor): A "serotonin-like" antidepressant with NE effects. It has a short half-life (less than 1 day rather than days), few side effects (nausea, sleepiness, dizziness and nervousness, sexual inhibition), and appears safe. Seems to be very promising (24). Aim for about 150 mg in divided doses, although it is also available in a slow-release form (Effexor XR). It appears to be particularly effective for *anxious depressions* and, in fact, may be effective for GAD itself. Withdrawal can be difficult.

Monoamine Oxidase Inhibitors

MAOIs are effective antidepressant/antipanic medications (25) and sometimes work when nothing else will, but due to their side effects, they are very rarely the drugs of first choice (Table 23.5). [In addition to the two drugs below, an additional "classic" MAOI discontinued several years ago has been released again by another company: isocarboxazid (Marplan).]

Indications for Use
Recommended for:

1. *Atypical depression*—An MAOI may be the drug of choice for "atypical depressions" (26) (50%–60% improve), i.e., depressed (F:M = 3–4:1) patients with varying degrees of (a) fatigue, anxious affect, rejection sensitivity, irritability, emotional lability, and/or (b) hyperphagia (often sweets), hypersomnolence, a "leaden feeling" in the limbs, reversed diurnal variation (worse in evening), and hypochondriasis. [Are there two types—anxious and vegetative (27)?] If a TCA or an SSRI is tried unsuccessfully, follow with a trial of an MAOI. ECT often fails with these patients.

Other uses:

- Patients with treatment-resistant (28) major depression (unipolar or bipolar) (29) or dysthymic disorder (30) and for whom ECT is not the obvious next choice.
- Panic disorder with or without agoraphobia (31) (particularly phenelzine; start slowly).
- Others: social phobia (32); PTSD (33); "perhaps" bulimia (use carefully in bingers).

Mechanisms of Action
MAOIs block MAO (and other enzymes) throughout the body (e.g., in blood, platelets, gut, CNS). MAO catalyzes the oxidation of such biogenic amines as NE, DA, 5-HT, and the amino acid tyramine. The therapeutic effect of MAOIs is *probably* related to the

TABLE 23.5 Monoamine Oxidase Inhibitors in Common Use (U.S.)

	Anti-cholinergic	Sedation	Dose (mg/day)	Starting dose
Phenelzine (Nardil)	1+	1+	30–90	15 mg t.i.d.
Tranylcypromine (Parnate)	1+	1+	20–60	10 mg b.i.d—t.i.d.

increase in CNS NE and 5-HT that results from the ability of MAOI to block oxidation of intracellular catecholamines.

MAO exists in two isoenzymes (34): MAO-A (in brain, liver, gut, and sympathetic nerves), which acts primarily on 5-HT and NE, and MAO-B (in brain, liver, and platelets), which acts on phenylethylamine and others. They both act on DA and tyramine. Also, the two available MAOIs (phenelzine, tranylcypromine) bind irreversibly to, and affect both types of, MAO. Due to the irreversibility, blood levels and drug half-life are of little importance: If you stop the MAOI, you must wait for new MAO to be synthesized (2 weeks) for the drug's effect to disappear.

No new MAOI antidepressants are available in the U.S., although the **RIMAs** (reversible inhibitors of monamine oxidase A) are being researched actively with *moclobemide* looking safe and possibly effective. Other specific MAOIs exist, such as: *clorgyline* (unavailable) inhibits MAO-A irreversibly; *pargyline* (Eutonyl—an antihypertensive) and *selegiline* (for Parkinson's disease) inhibit MAO-B; and *brofaromine* (unavailable), another RIMA. Safer, more specific, and effective MAOIs may be coming.

Pharmacokinetics

MAOIs are rapidly absorbed and are metabolized into inactive products (in hours) by several means, including acetylation (primarily phenelzine). There may be patients who are "rapid acetylators" and who require increased oral doses of MAOI. A clinical response usually takes 1–4 weeks. An 80%–90% inhibition of platelet MAO in blood samples seems necessary for clinical effectiveness (research measure).

Side Effects

MAOIs have numerous side effects. However, they lack the range of cardiotoxic effects of the TCAs, although some experts believe that they should be contraindicated in the elderly because of the risk of a potentially fatal hypertensive crisis (see below).

The most common side effects include drowsiness or stimulation (short lived), *insomnia* (10% or more of patients; often with suppression of REM sleep), dizziness, orthostatic *hypotension*, impotence (long-standing), urinary hesitancy, and weight gain (half of patients; mild but chronic). Dry mouth, constipation, and blurred vision are present but less of a problem than with TCAs due to minimal anticholinergic effects. MAOIs also can produce restlessness and irritability and can precipitate a manic episode. Up to 5% of patients have mildly elevated SGOT and SGPT; test further if malaise or jaundice develop.

A rare but potentially fatal side effect is the rapid onset of an ***hypertensive crisis*** (possible cerebrovascular bleeding and death) and hyperpyrexia in response to ingested tyramine (or other pressor amines). The MAO in the gut wall, which usually prevents entrance of large quantities of such ingested amines, is inhibited by MAOIs and thus a generalized sympathetic effect is allowed when tyramine-containing foods are eaten. The first sign of an impending crisis is usually a sudden severe occipital or temporal headache [followed/accompanied by sweating, nausea and vomiting, palpitations, restlessness, fever, neck stiffness, photophobia (dilated pupils), and rapidly rising BP] 20 minutes to 1 hour after eating. Patients (there is marked interindividual variation) taking MAOIs should avoid the italicized foods below completely and eat the other foods only in moderation (35):

- Protein-containing foods that are cultured or spoiled:
  Strong, aged cheeses (e.g., cheddar, blue, camembert, stilton)—cottage, ricotta, or cream cheeses are okay.
  Pickled or kippered herring; dried salted fish; snails; *shrimp paste.*
  Chicken livers (old livers of any kind) or *liver pate;* any *aged or slightly spoiled meat* (and *sausage, bologna, pepperoni, salami*); *protein extracts* and *protein dietary supplements.*
  Old yogurt, sour cream, chocolate (large amounts), licorice, *yeast* (except when used in baking).
- Nondistilled alcohol—red or *Chianti* wine (strict moderation); *vermouth;* beer [particularly *tap* (36) or *lager*]; coffee, tea, and colas.
- *Broad beans* (contain dopamine; e.g., Fava, Italian green, and lima beans); *bean curd, sauerkraut;* avocados; banana *peels;* soy sauce; soups prepared with bean curd or protein extracts (e.g., *miso soup*).

Treat a crisis with slow administration of phentolamine (Regitine, 5 mg IV); 0.25–0.5 mg IM q 4–6 hours later, if needed. It usually resolves in a few hours. The responsible patient may carry a 10-mg capsule of nifedipine (Procardia), bite it and place under the tongue, and then swallow for rapid relief when signs of a crisis appear (good for 3–6 hours; *visit an emergency room* because there is a risk of overshoot).

Drug Interactions
A number of adrenergic and sympathomimetic drugs may also produce serious interactions.

- *Hypertensive crisis*—Can be produced by amphetamines, cocaine, methylphenidate, and anorectics (stimulate NE release from adrenergic neurons), catecholamines (epinephrine, NE), sympathomimetic precursors (dopamine, methyldopa, levodopa), and sympathomimetic amines (ephedrine, phenylephrine, phenylpropanolamine, pseudoephedrine, metaraminol—check ingredients in over-the-counter cold, hay fever, and cough medication).
- Meperidine (Demerol)—Very dangerous combination. A few patients develop severe immediate hypertension, hyperpyrexia, and sweating *or* hypotension and coma. Narcotics may act similarly.
- CNS depression—Potentiated by alcohol, major tranquilizers, and hypnotic-sedatives.
- *Serotonin syndrome* (37) from conflicting antidepressants— Wait 2 weeks after stopping an SSRI, clomipramine, bupropion, nefazodone, or venlafaxine before starting an MAOI, and vice versa. Wait 5–6 weeks after stopping fluoxetine (*long* half-life of active metabolite norfluoxetine).

Treatment Principles
- Begin phenelzine 15 mg PO bid-tid and increase by 15 mg weekly to 60–90 mg/day. Maintain that dosage for 4 weeks before assuming a failure.
- Instruct the patient carefully about the potential side effects and which drugs and foods to avoid. Avoid using MAOIs in patients with pheochromocytoma or severe hypertension, renal disease, or liver disease.
- Maintenance is at acute treatment doses. In some patients, for unknown reasons, both the antidepressant and antiphobic effects become ineffective after 6 months to 1 year of use.
- Allow a 1–2 week washout before starting another drug; continue dietary restrictions for 2 weeks as well.

- If insomnia becomes a major problem, give all doses before mid-afternoon.
- Tranylcypromine is related to amphetamine and may have some stimulant properties.
- Do not give large prescriptions to impulsive, potentially suicidal outpatients.

Antidepressant Drug Combinations

Combined drug therapy may help a patient who has failed trials with single antidepressants. Such treatment is empirical (just about every conceivable combination has been tried by someone at some time). Proceed carefully and watch out for side effects (do *not* combine the SSRIs with the MAOIs). Potentially useful combinations include (38)

- **Antidepressant and lithium:** Probably the most effective mix for both unipolar and bipolar depression; adding lithium to a TCA or an MAOI occasionally may produce a *rapid* (days) improvement. Effective blood level varies from 0.4–1.0.
- **Antidepressant and antipsychotic:** For psychotic depressions.
- **Antidepressant and stimulant:** Used with TCAs or SSRIs; or use doses of dextroamphetamine, 5 mg tid or methylphenidate, 10 mg tid.
- **Antidepressant and thyroid:** Occasional patients improve (did they have a subclinical thyroid dysfunction?). Choose triiodothyronine (T_3), 25–50 µg/day; if ineffective, *stop*.
- **SSRI and TCA:** Literature is limited; clinical experience is more promising.
- **TCA or SSRIs and low-dose buspirone:** 10 mg tid (39).
- **Lithium or SSRI and bupropion:** For rapid cycling bipolars?

HYPNOTIC AND ANTIANXIETY DRUGS

Drugs Available

There are numerous drugs available for sedation, of which only the benzodiazepines and the new and unique agent buspirone can be recommended. Recognize that venlafaxine XR and perhaps several new antipsychotics may be useful antianxiety agents (Table 23.6).

TABLE 23.6 Sedative-Hypnotic Agents

Drug	Half-life (hr)	Dose (mg/day)
alprazolam (Xanax)	11–14	0.5–4
chlordiazepoxide (Librium)	15–60	15–60
clorazepate (Tranxene)	50–100	15–45
diazepam (Valium)	30–60	5–40
halazepam (Paxipam)	50–100	60–160
lorazepam (Ativan)	10–20	2–6
oxazepam (Serax)	5–10	30–120
prazepam (Centrax)	60–70	20–60
clonazepam (Klonopin)	30–40	1–4
estazolam (ProSom)	10–24	1–2 (HS)
flurazepam (Dalmane)	50 +	15–30 (HS)
quazepam (Doral)	40 +	7.5–15 (HS)
temazepam (Restoril)	8–18	15–30 (HS)
triazolam (Halcion)	2–3	0.125–0.25 (HS)
zaleplon (Sonata)	1–4	5–20 (HS)
zolpidem (Ambien)	2–3	5–10 (HS)
buspirone (Buspar)	2–3	15–60

Indications for Use

1. Short-term treatment of restlessness and anxiety (e.g., after life crises). They are *sedative at low dosage* and *hypnotic at higher doses.* They have no antipsychotic activity and thus should not be used as the exclusive treatment for psychotic disorders.
2. Generalized anxiety disorder and mild panic symptoms. Panic disorder (alprazolam, clonazepam).
3. Alcohol withdrawal (see Chapter 16); hypnotic-sedative withdrawal; psychosis due to hallucinogens.
4. Various seizure disorders.
5. Muscle relaxant (diazepam).

Mechanisms of Action and Pharmacokinetics

They enhance the inhibitory neurotransmitters (e.g., GABA, glycine) and have a specific depressant effect on the limbic system. As the dosage rises, there is generalized CNS depression. Buspirone, on the other hand, affects dopamine and serotonin receptors. They are well absorbed orally, are all both water and lipid soluble, and are usually metabolized by the liver but may also be excreted by the kidney. They are slowly and variably absorbed IM (faster by PO route). There is very little hepatic enzyme induc-

tion. Peak blood levels usually occur 1–4 hours after the oral dose
(1 hour for diazepam).

Side Effects

Compared with other classes of psychoactive drugs, side effects
are few.

- Most common problem is CNS depression manifested by
  daytime sedation, decreased concentration, and poor coordination in some patients at therapeutic doses. They are
  very safe drugs, although a massive OD or combination with
  alcohol or other drugs will produce life-threatening CNS
  depression.
- Anterograde amnesia can occur after hypnotic-induced sleep
  with short-acting drugs (e.g., lorazepam, triazolam). Patients
  may lose memory for events that occurred during the night *or*
  during the following day.
- Tolerance and physical addiction occur, particularly with
  short-acting drugs or when taken at high doses for several
  months. The withdrawal syndrome is usually mild (but may be
  severe: rebound anxiety, nausea, sweating, hyperalertness,
  and occasionally seizures) and typically occurs 2–14 days
  after stopping the drug (most rapid with the shorter acting drugs). Discontinuing alprazolam may be particularly
  difficult (withdrawal symptoms can include paranoia,
  marked anxiety and agitation, psychosis, hallucinations, and
  seizures)—go *very* slowly (e.g., decrease 0.5 mg weekly at first,
  then 0.25 mg weekly below a total daily dose of 2 mg).
- Untoward but infrequent psychiatric manifestations include
  exacerbation of schizophrenia and depression.
- There appear to be *no* autonomic side effects.
- Benzodiazepines seem to be safe in pregnancy.

Drug Interactions

- There is an increased sedative effect when combined with
  CNS depressants (e.g., alcohol). Moreover, the combination
  with alcohol at times actually may be anxiogenic.
- Disulfiram (Antabuse) and cimetidine impair the metabolism
  of the long-acting benzodiazepines and thus raise the plasma
  levels. The shorter-acting drugs appear less affected.

- Food, antacids, and anticholinergic drugs appear to decrease the rate, but not the extent, of drug absorption.

Treatment Principles

- Use the long-acting benzodiazepines (chlordiazepoxide, diazepam, clorazepate) on an HS or bid schedule. Use a tid-qid schedule for the shorter acting ones (oxazepam, lorazepam).
- Recognize that the longer acting drugs (and their active metabolites) may accumulate over days or weeks, producing increasing symptoms of sedation. Lorazepam and oxazepam have a simple metabolism and do not accumulate.
- Try to avoid use for longer than 1–3 weeks in most patients either as a sedative or a hypnotic. Some patients may be able to use them less frequently but on a long-term, "as needed" basis, but be alert for those patients prone to abuse. Reevaluate if you find that you have used medication for longer than 2–4 months (however, a few patients seem to do well on *low* doses for long periods—not recommended if it can be avoided). Addiction can occur (particularly among alcoholics) but is uncommon.
- Use by PO route, if possible.
- Encourage the patient to avoid the simultaneous use of a benzodiazepine and alcohol or another sedative-hypnotic drug.
- Be *very* careful when giving to the elderly—confusion is common. Dosage may need to be 20% or less of the usual young adult dose.
- If the patient has been taking benzodiazepines for several months, stop medication over 2–3 weeks (particularly the long-acting drugs).
- The more sedative benzodiazepines and those with shorter half-lives are used primarily as hypnotics, although in adequate dosage any drug in this class can be hypnotic. Flurazepam is rapidly absorbed and is useful for sleep onset problems; temazepam and flurazepam may help frequent awakening. Flurazepam, particularly because of its long-acting metabolite *N*-desalkylflurazepam (quazepam has the same major active metabolite) accumulates and produces a hangover in a few (often older) patients. Triazolam is very short-acting and does not accumulate but has been associated in a number of

patients with "withdrawal-like" symptoms after each dose, e.g., early morning insomnia, irritability, daytime anxiety and dysphoria [and even (rare) confusion and paranoia]. (It has been "accused" of producing rage attacks in some patients; the issue remains unsettled but the drug looks suspicious.)

- Zolpidem (Ambien; rapidly absorbed, short half-life, minimal rebound insomnia or daytime somnolence) is a new non-benzodiazepine hypnotic that may be an improvement but may have the usual problems of tolerance with extended use and addiction at higher doses. A second new hypnotic is zaleplon (Sonata rapidly absorbed; short half-life; affects the $GABA_A$; receptor complex) that is most like triazolam and zolpidem and appears to share their problems as well.

Buspirone represents a new class of anxiolytics [a serotonin (5-HT_{1A}) agonist]. It has few side effects, produces less sedation and cognitive and psychomotor impairment than the benzodiazepines, is not likely to be abused, but may be less effective as well. It is a reasonable alternative drug, particularly for chronic anxiety states and in the elderly. Begin at 5 mg tid (5 mg/day in the elderly) and increase over 10 days to the average daily dose of 20–30 mg, bid-tid. Unlike the benzodiazepines, expect 2–3 weeks before it begins to work. It "may" also augment the antidepressant effects of the SSRIs and decrease agitation in the demented elderly.

PSYCHOTROPIC MEDICATION USE DURING PREGNANCY

In general, the absolute risk on the infant of a mother's use of psychotropic medication during pregnancy is low (40). In most cases (e.g., even in the notorious situation of using Li to control mania in the pregnant woman) the treated condition is much safer for the infant (41). This topic suffers from a general lack of knowledge about the effects of most medications, particularly the newer drugs. Most information comes either from animal studies or, after release of a medication, in women discovered to have become pregnant while taking the drug.

The most conservative approach is to avoid any medication not proven safe. This is almost certainly unnecessarily cautious. The risk-to-benefit ratio would suggest that most medication should be used (with care) if needed. No psychotropic medication has been shown to be seriously dangerous to the infant. The "short list" of those medications that generally should be avoided (unless truly needed) includes (42) lithium (due to rare cardiovascular anomalies), fluoxetine (maybe) in the third trimester, valproic acid and carbamazepine in the first trimester due to 1%–2% incidence of neural tube defects, diazepam and several other benzodiazepines due to an infrequent oral cleft defect (clonazepam and lorazepam seem to be okay), and benzodiazepine hypnotics just on general principles. Interestingly, clozapine seems to be safe.

ELECTROCONVULSIVE THERAPY

Despite its unjustified notoriety, ECT is legitimate. Although its mechanism of action is unknown, it is effective, painless, and safe (mortality rate less than competing therapies or the untreated state: 0.01%–0.03% of patients treated—mostly cardiovascular deaths). However, before administration *always* obtain

1. Informed consent from a voluntary, competent patient.
2. Informed consent from a relative or guardian of a voluntary, incompetent patient and an independent psychiatric opinion of therapeutic need.
3. Court approval for administration to a resisting, involuntary patient who is a danger to him or herself or others.

Discuss the risks of amnesia, confusion, and headache with the patient and his or her family. Also discuss the risks of *not* receiving ECT.

Indications for Use

ECT is a serious procedure; use *only* in those conditions for which it is recommended. It is tempting to give ECT to any patient who is not improving—do not!

- **Major affective illness:** Patients with *major depression* or *bipolar disorder, depressed* respond well to ECT (80%–90% recover vs. 70% or more treated with antidepressants). Patients with marked vegetative symptoms (e.g., insomnia, constipation, suicidal rumination, obsessions with guilt, anorexia and weight loss, psychomotor retardation) are particularly responsive. ECT is much more effective than antidepressants for psychotically depressed patients (i.e., vegetative symptoms and paranoid or somatic delusions). Give antidepressants a full trial (e.g., imipramine 200–300 mg/day for 4 weeks) and then con-

sider ECT if there is no improvement. Mania (*bipolar disorder, manic*) also responds to ECT; typically used only if lithium carbonate (+ antipsychotic) fails to control the acute phase.
- Schizophrenic disorders: *Catatonic schizophrenia* of either stuporous or excited type responds well to ECT. Try antipsychotic medication first, but if the condition is life-threatening (e.g., hyperexcited delirium), go quickly to ECT. Occasional acutely psychotic patients (particularly of the schizoaffective type) who do not respond to medication alone may improve if ECT is added, but for most schizophrenics (e.g., chronics) it is of little value.

ECT is the *treatment of choice* for

1. Actively suicidal depressed patients who may not live until antidepressants begin to work.
2. Depressed patients (particularly the elderly) whose medical condition makes administration of antidepressants risky. Patients with both depression and OBS may do better with ECT. ECT *can* be safely performed during pregnancy.
3. Seriously depressed patients who have had an *adequate* trial of antidepressants (60%–70% recovers with ECT).

Contraindications for Use

There are no *absolute* contraindications. Always weigh the risk of the procedure against the danger incurred if the patient is untreated. Neurologic disease is not a contraindication. Response improves with age; patients under 30 respond more poorly.

- *Very high risk:*
  Increased intracranial pressure (e.g., brain tumor, CNS infection): ECT briefly increases CSF pressure and risks tentorial herniation. Always check for papilledema before administration.
  Recent MI: ECT frequently causes arrhythmias (vagal arrhythmias producing postictal PVCs and extravagal arrhythmias producing PVCs anytime during the procedure) that can be fatal if there has been recent muscle damage. Wait until enzymes and ECG have stabilized.
- *Moderate risk:*
  Severe osteoarthritis, osteoporosis, or recent fracture: Prepare thoroughly for treatment (i.e., with muscle relaxants); retinal detachment.

Cardiovascular disease (e.g., hypertension, angina, aneurysm, arrhythmias): Premedicate carefully; have a cardiologist available.

Major infections, recent CVA, chronic respiratory difficulty, acute peptic ulcer, pheochromocytoma.

Techniques of Administration

Pre-ECT Medical Workup:
Complete history and physical, concentrating on cardiac and neurologic status, CBC, chemistry, UA, VDRL, chest and spine x-rays, ECG. Get EEG (and/or CT scan) if neurologic is abnormal.

A Typical Technique:
ECT routines vary—there is no "one right way." Usually perform in a hospital and with the aid of an anesthesiologist.

1. Prepare the patient with information and psychological support. Have him or her void and defecate beforehand. NPO after midnight. If markedly anxious, give 5 mg of diazepam IM 1–2 hours before treatment. Antidepressants, antipsychotics, sedative-hypnotics, and anticonvulsants (among others) should be stopped the day before treatment. Lithium usually should be stopped several days beforehand; risk is organicity.

2. Make patient comfortable. Remove dentures. Hyperextend the back with a pillow.

3. When ready, premedicate with atropine (0.6–1.2 mg SC, IM, or IV). This anticholinergic controls vagal arrhythmias and reduces GI secretions.

4. Provide 90%–100% oxygen by bag when respirations are not spontaneous.

5. Give sodium *methohexital* (Brevital) (40–100 mg IV, rapidly). This short-acting barbiturate anesthetic is used to produce a light coma.

6. Next, quickly give enough of the muscle relaxant *succinylcholine* (Anectine) (30–80 mg IV, rapidly—monitor depth of relaxation by the muscle fasciculations produced) to remove all but very minor evidences of a generalized seizure (e.g., plantarflexion).

7. Once relaxed, place a bite block in the mouth and then give electroconvulsive stimulus. Two methods are common and acceptable today:

   Unilateral: One electrode placed in the frontotemporal area and the other 7–10 cm away in the parietal region—both on the nondominant hemisphere (right side for right-handed persons, 60% R and 40% L for left-handers). Unilateral ECT is commonly used because it produces less postictal confusion and amnesia but it seems to be less effective than bilateral ECT.

   Bilateral: Bifrontotemporal electrode placement. This is the traditional technique—effective but produces more side effects (e.g., amnesia, headache).

   Effectiveness of either method depends on producing a central generalized seizure (peripheral effects are not necessary) lasting at least 25 seconds. Monitor this with EEG, peripheral EMG, or the tonic/clonic movement of the hand on the same side as the electrode (unilateral) that has been freed of muscle relaxant by a tight cuff applied before the administration of the succinylcholine. If a seizure is not produced, increase the stimulus and repeat ("missed" or unilateral seizures are usually of little therapeutic value; they occur more frequently with unilateral shock, perhaps accounting for its lesser effectiveness).

8. Monitor patient carefully until stable—there is usually 15–30 minutes of postictal confusion. These patients are at risk for prolonged apnea and a postictal delirium (5–10 mg of IV diazepam may help).

Complications of ECT

- Amnesia (retrograde and anterograde)—Variable; beginning after 3–4 treatments; lasting weeks to 2–3 months (but occasionally much longer); more severe with bilateral placement, increased number of treatments, increased current strength, and prior presence of organicity.
- Headache, muscle aches, nausea.
- Dizziness, confusion—The persistence and severity of the confusion increases with an increasing number of treatments.
- Reserpine and ECT given concurrently have resulted in fatalities.

- Fractures—Rare with good muscle relaxation.
- ECT anesthesia risks:
  Atropine worsens narrow angle glaucoma.
  Succinylcholine's action is prolonged in pseudocholinesterase deficiency states. These conditions (malnutrition, liver disease, chronic renal dialysis, use of echothiophate for glaucoma) can lead to potentially fatal hypotonia.
  Procainamide, lidocaine, and quinidine can potentiate succinylcholine.
  Methohexital can precipitate an attack of acute intermittent porphyria.

Treatment Principles

1. Usually give one treatment per day on alternate days.
2. Depressions usually require 6–12 treatments. Mania and catatonia require 10–20. Expect to see improved behavior after 2–6 treatments if it is going to be effective. Allow the clinical response to determine the treatment end point. Be *very cautious* (and seek a second opinion) about exceeding 20 treatments during one period of illness.
3. Maintenance ECT (single treatments every 1–3 months during the months or years after recovery) *may* be useful, particularly with elderly depressed patients, but should be used primarily if medication is contraindicated.
4. Maintenance antidepressants, antipsychotics, and lithium (begun after a successful course of ECT) may forestall relapse. Without medication, the relapse rate is high.

PSYCHOSURGERY

Little psychosurgery is currently performed in the United States. Modern psychosurgeons make one of several possible small cuts in the brain (usually in the limbic system) that can improve a variety of psychiatric conditions and that have few side effects (unlike the widely destructive prefrontal lobotomy of the past).

All candidates for surgery must have an intractable and devastating condition unrelieved by any other therapy. Conditions likely to respond include chronic pain with depression and severe depression alone. Improvement occurs in some patients who have severe obsessive-compulsive and anxiety states and in a few schizophrenics. The mechanism for the improvement is uncertain, and a variety of different surgical cuts yield similar results. Despite the lack of theoretic sophistication, there are patients for whom psychosurgery is a valid "last resort."

REFERENCES

1. Schatzberg AF, Nemeroff CB. *Textbook of psychopharmacology,* 2nd ed. Washington, DC: American Psychiatric Press, 1998.
2. Risch SC. Pathophysiology of schizophrenia and the role of newer antipsychotics. *Pharmacotherapy* 1996;16:11–14.
3. Osser DN, Zarate CA. Consultant for the pharmacotherapy of schizophrenia. *Psychiatric Ann* 1999;29:252–267.
4. Conley RR, Tamminga CA, Bartko JJ, et al. Olanzapine compared with chlorpromazine in treatment-resistant schizophrenia. *Am J Psychiatry* 1998;155:914–920.
5. Franz M, Lis S, Plüddemann, et al. Conventional versus atypical neuroleptics: subjective quality of life in schizophrenic patients. *Br J Psychiatry* 1997;170:422–425.
6. Conley RR, Love RC, Kelly DL, et al. Rehospitalization rates of patients recently discharged on a regimen of risperidone or clozapine. *Am J Psychiatry* 1999;156:863–868.
7. Bradford DW, Chakos MH, Sheitman BB, et al. Atypical antipsychotic drugs in treatment-refractory schizophrenia. *Psychiatric Ann* 1998;28:618–626.
8. Simpson GM, Lindenmayer J. Extrapyramidal symptoms in patients treated with risperidone. *J Clin Psychopharmacol* 1997;17:194–201.
9. Grof P. Has the effectiveness of lithium changed? *Neuropsychopharmacology* 1998;19:183–188.
10. Faedda GL, Tondo L, Baldessarini RJ: Outcome after rapid vs. gradual discontinuation of lithium treatment in bipolar disorders. *Arch Gen Psychiatry* 1993;50:448–455.
11. Johnson G. Lithium—early development, toxicity, and renal function. *Neuropsychopharmacology* 1998;19:200–205.
12. Dunn RT, Frye MS, Kimbrell TA, et al. The efficacy and use of anticonvulsants in mood disorders. *Clin Neuropharmacol* 1998;21:215–235.
13. Freeman MP, Stoll AL. Mood stabilizer combinations: a review of safety and efficacy. *Am J Psychiatry* 1998;155:12–21.
14. Bowden CL, Janicak PG, Orsulak P, et al. Relation of serum valproate concentration to response in mania. *Am J Psychiatry* 1996;153:765–770.
15. Kotler M, Matar MA. Lamotrigine in the treatment of resistant bipolar disorder. *Clin Neuropharmacol* 1998;21:65–67.

16. Erfurth A, Kammerer C, Grunze H, et al. An open label study of gabapentin in the treatment of acute mania. *J Psychiatric Res* 1998;32: 261–264.

17. Calabrese JR, Kimmel SE, Woyshville MJ, et al. Clozapine for treatment-refractory mania. *Am J Psychiatry* 1996;153:759–764.

18. Segal J, Berk M, Brook S. Risperidone compared with both lithium and haloperidol in mania. *Clin Neuropharmacol* 1998;21:176–180.

19. McElroy SL, Frye M, Denicoff K, et al. Olanzapine in treatment-resistant bipolar disorder. *J Affect Disord* 1998;49:119–122.

20. Zanardi R, Franchini L, Gasperini M, et al. Double-blind controlled trial of sertraline versus paroxetine in the treatment of delusional depression. *Am J Psychiatry* 1996;153:1631–1633.

21. Gatti F, Bellini L, Gasperini M, et al. Fluvoxamine alone in the treatment of delusional depression. *Am J Psychiatry* 1996;153:414–416.

22. Burrows GD, Maguire KP, Norman TR. Antidepressant efficacy and tolerability of the selective norepinephrine reuptake inhibitor reboxetine: a review. *J Clin Psychiatry* 1998;59[Suppl 14]:4–7.

23. Lane R, Baldwin D. Selective serotonin reuptake inhibitor-induced serotonin syndrome: review. *J Clin Psychopharmacol* 1997;17:208–221.

24. Benkert O, Gründer G, Wetzel H. Is there an advantage to venlafaxine in comparison with other antidepressants? *Hum Psychopharmacol* 1997;12: 53–64.

25. Thase ME, Trivedi MH, Rush AJ. MAOIs in contemporary treatment of depression. *Neuropsychopharmacology* 1995;12:185–219.

26. Quitkin FM, Harrison W, Stewart JW, et al. Response to phenelzine and imipramine in placebo nonresponders with atypical depression: a new application of the crossover design. *Arch Gen Psychiatry* 1991; 48:319–323.

27. Davidson J, Pelton S. Forms of atypical depression and their response to antidepressant drugs. *Psychiatric Res* 1986;17:87–93.

28. Thase ME, Frank E, Mallinger AG, et al. Treatment of imipramine-resistant recurrent depression. III. Efficacy of monamine oxidase inhibitors. *J Clin Psychiatry* 1992;53:5–11.

29. Himmelhoch JM, Thase ME, Mallinger AG, et al. Tranylcypromine versus imipramine in anergic bipolar depression. *Am J Psychiatry* 1991;148:910–916.

30. Howland RH. Pharmacotherapy of dysthymia: a review. *J Clin Psychopharmacol* 1991;11:83–92.

31. Jefferson JW. Antidepressants in panic disorder. *J Clin Psychiatry* 1992;58[Suppl 2]:20–24.

32. Den-Boer JA, van-Vliet IM, Westenberg HG. Recent developments in the psychopharmacology of social phobia. *Eur Arch Psychiatry Clin Neurosci* 1995;244:309–316.

33. Davidson JR. Biological therapies for posttraumatic stress disorder: an overview. *J Clin Psychiatry* 1997;58[Suppl 9]:29–32.

34. Cesura AM, Pletscher A. The new generations of monoamine oxidase inhibitors. *Prog Drug Res* 1992;38:171–297.

35. Gardner DM, Shulman KI, Walker SE, et al. The making of a user friendly MAOI diet. *J Clin Psychiatry* 1996;57:99–104.

36. Shulman KI, Tailor SA, Walker SE, et al. Tap (draft) beer and monoamine oxidase inhibitor dietary restrictions. *Can J Psychiatry* 1997;42:310–312.

37. Bodner RA, Lynch T, Lewis L, et al. Serotonin syndrome. *Neurology* 1995;45:219–223.

38. Nelson JC. Treatment of antidepressant nonresponders: augmentation or switch? *J Clin Psychiatry* 1998;59[Suppl 15]:35–41.

39. Dimitriou EC, Dimitriou CE. Buspirone augmentation of antidepressant therapy. *J Clin Psychopharmacol* 1998;18:465–469.

40. Altshuler LL, Cohen LS, Szuba MP, et al. Pharmacologic management of psychiatric illness during pregnancy. *Am J Psychiatry* 1996;153:592–606.

41. Cohen LS, Friedman JM, Jefferson JW, et al. A reevaluation of risk of in utero exposure to lithium. *JAMA* 1994;271:146–150.

42. Barki ZHK, Kravitz HM, Berki TM. Psychotropic medications in pregnancy. *Psychiatric Ann* 1998;28:486–500.

Chapter 24

The Elderly Patient

More than 25,000,000 Americans are over 65: 85% have a chronic illness (usually medical) and 20%–30% have a psychiatric illness (most common in the very old) (1,2).

EVALUATION OF THE ELDERLY

1. Assess each patient carefully—mental decline is *not* normal for the aged.
2. Always carefully evaluate physical condition. An impaired physical state can markedly alter the psychiatric evaluation. Make sure the patient can hear and see. Check for deficiency states (iron, folate, vitamins B_{12} and D, calcium, serum proteins).
3. Interview technique: Be respectful, use surname, sit near, speak slowly and clearly, allow time for answers, be friendly and personal, pat and hug, be supportive and issue oriented, keep interview short.
4. Collect history, do mental status—Perhaps in more than one interview.
5. Identify premorbid personality—Defense mechanisms and coping styles (e.g., independent vs. passive–dependent, rigid vs. flexible, use of denial, etc.).
6. Assess the major *risk factors:*
   a. Loss—of spouse, friends, physical health, job, status, independence, etc.
   b. Poverty—many elderly are poor; some are victims of crime.

    c. Social isolation—impaired mobility, few friends, etc.
    d. Sensory deprivation—poor hearing, vision, etc.
    e. Sickness—chronic pain, forced inactivity, etc.
    f. Fears—of being dependent, of being alone, of being helpless.
7. See family—Assess their strengths, dynamics, support for the patient, hidden agendas.

COMMON PSYCHIATRIC DISORDERS

Delirium

Common and commonly overlooked or mistaken for depression (3). May be the primary presentation of

1. CNS—Cerebral infarction (embolic or thrombotic), TIAs, neoplasms.
2. Heart—MI (often without pain), arrhythmia, CHF.
3. Lungs—Pneumonia (without fever or leukocytosis), PE (without chest pain, dyspnea, tachycardia).
4. Blood—Anemia.
5. Metabolic—Diabetes, liver failure, hyper- or hypothyroidism, electrolyte abnormalities.
6. Psychogenic—Strange surroundings, stress.
7. Infections—Most kinds.
8. Other—Medication reaction, *alcoholism,* prescription drug misuse, dehydration, fecal impaction, "silent" appendicitis, urinary retention, UTIs, eye or ear disease, postoperative.

Treat the underlying disease process, if possible. Keep patient in a lighted room and with familiar surroundings and people. Restrain only if essential. If needed, use small doses of major tranquilizers (e.g., thioridazine 25–50 mg PO, often given as an HS dose; thiothixene 2–5 mg PO or 4 mg IM). Mild delirium may continue (unnoticed) for months after the acute episode.

Dementia

Most elderly have unimpaired intellectual functioning. Dementia (20% of those 80 years old) is not "just a result of aging"; it needs an explanation. Dementia often presents first with agitation, anxiety, depression, and/or somatic complaints. *Always* do a mental status examination on elderly patients with these complaints, but remember that it can also be mimicked by depression, serious physical conditions, alcoholism, and malnutrition. Dementia in the elderly frequently occurs with and is made worse by depression or delirium. Treat the agitated demented patient with low-dose neuroleptics or benzodiazepines initially, then after several weeks, switch to SSRIs, buspirone, and/or trazadone; or later consider beta-blockers. Marked memory loss may be unrecognized by the patient but is of major concern to the family, who ultimately insist on evaluation and treatment for it.

Most patients with a progressive and nonreversible form of dementia can be maintained at home until the late stages of the disease process. The decision to institutionalize depends not only on what facilities are available locally (some may be very good) but also on the realistic strengths and limits of the family. Once the cause and prognosis of the dementia is determined, the physician may most profitably spend his or her time helping the family draw limits, handle guilt, and adjust.

Depression

Major depression can develop in old age for the first time or be a recurrence of a major affective disorder. In the elderly it may at times closely mimic a dementia (pseudodementia); or physical symptoms, apathy, or fatigue may dominate the clinical picture. It is common, frequently unrecognized, often has a long course compared with that of a younger person, is potentially fatal (both from physical inanition and from suicide; remember, the highest suicide rate is among elderly males, particularly with alcoholism), and responds well to treatment. Several recent studies tie its presence very closely to subtle cerebrovascular disease (4–7). When in doubt, hospitalize. Treat first with psychotherapy and then, particularly if severe, with antidepressants (increase slowly; effective final daily oral dose may be as low as 10–50 mg of nortriptyline or 10 mg of fluoxetine). Consider low-dose SSRI as an appropriate first-line medication. ECT may be the therapy of choice in patients with unstable cardiac status or in those patients with psychotic depression (e.g., paranoia, hallucinations).

A less severe depression or depressive equivalent (listlessness, physical complaints, withdrawal) in a patient with long-standing depressive complaints may represent *dysthymic disorder*

(8). Because stress and loss are so common among the elderly, *adjustment disorder with depressed mood* and *bereavement* occur frequently.

Other Disorders

Mania (9) does occur in old age but usually with a history of bipolar disorder. Extreme agitation or manic-like behavior can be caused by organic factors, dementia, schizophrenia, depression, or situational anxiety. Lithium and anticonvulsants are effective.

Schizophrenia usually has a life-long history, but rarely the stresses of old age can precipitate a first episode in a predisposed individual (long-standing schizoid or borderline functioning). Occasionally there is associated intellectual deterioration. Treat with support and antipsychotics.

Paranoia or mild suspiciousness among the elderly is very common (10). Bizarre forms or near psychotic levels may occur with

1. Early dementia—*always* check for intellectual loss;
2. Delirium;
3. Vision or hearing problems—may resolve promptly;
4. Social isolation; chronic illness;
5. Drugs—e.g., steroids, antiparkinsonians, hypnotic withdrawal.

DELUSIONAL DISORDER (DSM-IV p. 301, 297.1) often has an onset late in life (late-life paraphrenia). These patients have fixed paranoid delusions and occasionally auditory hallucinations but not the loose associations, grandiosity, major hallucinations, and autistic thought of paranoid schizophrenics (although the conditions may overlap). Treat with reality-oriented psychotherapy, behavior modification, maintenance antipsychotics, and possibly ECT.

Hypochondriasis

The elderly are frequently ill and may develop a preoccupation with exaggerated physical complaints and problems. This is particularly common among depressed and/or demented elderly. The physical symptoms may or may not improve with resolution of the depression.

The patient with severe hypochondriasis, whose life is dominated by ruminations about one or more physical problems, is very difficult to treat. Withdrawal and isolation are frequent. Do not expect a "cure." Develop an ongoing relationship with this patient. Be available. See every 2–3 weeks for 10–20 minutes. Reassure that the problem may be persistent and incurable but not debilitating or fatal. Recognize that in some cases symptoms may continue because to lose them would mean to lose the reason for visiting the physician.

Adjustment Disorders

These are common in old age and are due to the numerous stresses (loss, physical illness, retirement, etc.) encountered. Symptoms include anxiety, depression, agitation, and physical complaints and most often occur in persons with past adjustment problems. Grief is common and may mimic a major depression but often has an obvious precipitant, is short-lived with therapy, and does not require antidepressants. *Alcohol abuse* is also a common response to stress in the elderly and is frequently unrecognized. Supportive psychotherapy, attention to concrete problems, and brief use of minor tranquilizers or low-dose antipsychotics helps.

PSYCHOPHARMACOLOGY OF OLD AGE

The elderly usually run higher blood levels (due to decreased hepatic metabolism and renal excretion, reduced plasma albumin and protein binding, and increased fat to lean tissue ratios), display increased receptor responsiveness, and thus require more gradual increases and *lower doses* of most psychoactive medication. They are also more susceptible to most side effects (e.g., peripheral and central anticholinergic effects, sedation, hypotension, arrhythmias). They are at risk for bowel obstruction, urinary retention, BP problems (fainting, stroke), sudden death from fatal arrhythmias, glaucoma crises, delirium, and coma. Also, they are particularly likely to be taking multiple drugs, to misunderstand and fail to comply with prescribing instruction, and to have symptoms from such polypharmacy. Preferable medication for the elderly include

- **Benzodiazepines:** For anxiety, oxazepam (15–30 mg/day) and lorazepam (0.5–3 mg/day) are least likely to accumulate. Venlafaxine XR is expensive but effective; buspirone is slightly less effective but very safe. In patients with insomnia, try relaxation or exercise first. If a medication is needed, try temazepam (7.5–15 mg HS; limited accumulation) or zolpidem (2.5–5 mg HS).

- **Antidepressants:** Low doses of the SSRIs and other newer antidepressants have become the drugs of choice. TCAs and even MAOIs can be used, but secondarily and cautiously (i.e., effective but too many side effects).
- **Antipsychotics:** Usually choose the more potent least sedating types (e.g., haloperidol, trifluoperazine) but be guided by patient's side effects. With IM meds, consider U-100 insulin syringes to ensure a small dose. Small doses of the new antipsychotics (e.g., risperidone, olanzapine) are soon likely to be the medications of choice.
- **Lithium:** Toxicity occurs easily, so keep on a lower maintenance level (e.g., 0.4–0.7 mEq/L).

GENERAL TREATMENT PRINCIPLES

- Be *supportive,* respectful, sympathetic, and a "good listener." Touch the patient.
- Encourage patients to express themselves (about guilt, loneliness, helplessness) and unburden themselves (e.g., grieve).
- Be directive and reality oriented. Help in a concrete way with problems (e.g., who to see about rent assistance, calling "Meals-on-Wheels," explanation of Medicare benefits). The quality of the patient's current environment is probably the single most important factor promoting recovery and continued health.
- Strengthen defenses rather than restructure them.
- Encourage self-esteem. Helping patients "review their life" (to see it as complete) can be enormously beneficial. Reminiscence *is* adaptive coping behavior and helps promote self-esteem.
- Encourage continued interests, friendships, socialization, activities, and self-support. Identify those things still done well and encourage the patient to continue to do them (if they cannot fix the meal, maybe they can still set the table).
- Be an ongoing presence. Be available—frequent, regular, short sessions. Be reachable by telephone.
- Involve and work with the family. Teach them appropriate skills and expectation. Anger, frustrations, and resentment often develop—help them deal with these feelings.

- A psychotherapy group of elderly patients is often very helpful—locate one for the patient.
- Know and use community resources.

REFERENCES

1. Jenike MA. Psychiatric illnesses in the elderly: a review. *J Geriatr Psychiatry Neurol* 1996;9:57–82.
2. Sadavoy J, Lazarus LW, Jarvik LF, et al. *Comprehensive review of geriatric psychiatry,* 2nd ed. Washington, DC: American Psychiatric Press, 1996.
3. Farrell KR, Ganzini L. Misdiagnosing delirium as depression in medically ill elderly patients. *Arch Intern Med* 1995;155:2459–2464.
4. Greenwald BS, Kramer-Ginsberg E, Krishnan KRR, et al. MRI signal hyperintensities in geriatric depression. *Am J Psychiatry* 1996;153:1212–1215.
5. Lawlor BA, Anderson MC. The neurobiology of late-life depression: impact of silent cerebrovascular disease. *Hum Psychopharmacol* 1995;10:S223–S227.
6. Lesser IM, Boone KB, Mehringer CM, et al. Cognition and white matter hyperintensities in older depressed patients. *Am J Psychiatry* 1996;153:1280–1287.
7. Salloway S, Malloy P, Kohn R, et al. MRI and neuropsychological differences in early- and late-life-onset geriatric depression. *Neurology* 1996;46:1567–1574.
8. Weiss KJ. Management of anxiety and depression syndromes in the elderly. *J Clin Psychiatry* 1994;55[Suppl 2]:5–12.
9. Chen ST, Altshuler LL, Spar JE. Bipolar disorder in late life: a review. *J Geriatr Psychiatry Neurol* 1998;11:29–35.
10. Holden NL. Late paraphrenia or the paraphrenias? *Br J Psychiatry* 1987;150:635–639.

Chapter 25

Legal Issues

The interface between psychiatry and law is in flux, partly due to recent patient's rights legislation (based on the constitutional assurance that no person shall be deprived of his or her liberty without "due process of law") (1,2). A psychiatrist's dealings with his or her patients increasingly are constrained by case law and statue. It is essential that he or she learn the limits to their independence. Laws can differ markedly from state to state and may change with time—become familiar with those laws that apply to your area.

CIVIL LAW

Civil Commitment

All states permit civil commitment to inpatient (and, at times, outpatient) psychiatric care under specific, but differing, criteria. Know your local standards.

1. **Mental Illness:** All states require the presence of a mental illness, but definitions differ (3). Psychosis usually is included, but personality disorder is not. Drug and/or alcohol abuse may be allowed. Mental illness alone is not sufficient for commitment but requires at least one of the following two additional conditions.
2. **Dangerousness:** To self or others: Most states require that the patient be dangerous but differ in the degree of urgency—an *imminent* danger (e.g., likely to hurt him or herself in the next 24 hours) versus a relative danger (e.g., physically deteriorat-

ing through depressive withdrawal). Dangerousness is the most common reason for commitment in most states. Two major problems with the dangerousness standard are (a) psychiatrists have difficulty accurately predicting future dangerous behavior except in the most obvious cases and (b) it has been uncertain what level of proof the law requires—i.e., from the lowest civil standard of "preponderance of the evidence" (51% certainty) to the most strict criminal standard of "beyond a reasonable doubt" (95% certainty). This latter issue appears to have been resolved by a recent U.S. Supreme Court decision (*Addington v Texas,* 1979) favoring "clear and convincing evidence" (75% certainty).

3. **Disabled and in need of treatment:** Although diminished in degree, most states allow commitment solely on the grounds that a person is significantly handicapped by a mental illness, is unable to provide for his or her own basic needs (the *parens patriae* provision), and is in need of, and would benefit from, treatment.

Most states also have laws (usually less strict) allowing the patient to be briefly (1–14 days) held involuntarily (4). There recently has been a growing tendency in the law toward "a duty to commit" worrisome patients (*Schuster v Altenberg,* 1988). Committed patients who believe they are being held illegally may obtain a hearing by a *writ of habeas corpus.*

Much recent legislation defining these standards has redressed real past wrongs that occurred when commitment could result merely from a physician's "okay," yet recent controversy has focused on associated losses to the patient and their family due to his or her exclusion from treatment because of complex criminal-like commitment proceedings. As fewer patients have been treated involuntarily, some experts have noted a shift of mental patients from the civil to the criminal system—i.e., the mental illness *causes* them to break a law they ordinarily would not have broken and they are then arrested. The extent of this trend remains undetermined.

An additional impact of the changing commitment laws has been to require the release of committed patients much earlier than in the past, resulting in a marked decline in the size of state mental hospitals. An unfortunate effect of this deinstitutionalization has been to release large numbers of marginally functional persons into communities ill equipped to deal with them, with the resultant formation of "psychiatric ghettos" in some large cities.

The Right to Treatment

Following the classic Alabama decision of *Wyatt v Stickney* (1972), it has become a general standard (amazingly, it had not been before) that an involuntarily committed person must receive a level of effective treatment adequate to encourage improvement. This concept was challenged, reviewed, and supported in another well-known case—*Donaldson v O'Connor* (1974). How to deal with the patient who is unlikely to improve with *any* treatment remains uncertain (5).

The Right to Refuse Treatment

This is currently one of the most actively contested areas of psychiatric law, and the results of the debate remain uncertain. Involuntary commitment is *not* prima facie evidence that the patient is incompetent to decide what treatment he or she is to receive. Federal court decisions set the tone but conflict: *Rennie v Klein* (1979) gives a patient a qualified right to refuse treatment and creates an appeal process, whereas *Rogers v Okin* (1981) allows absolute refusal but provides for treatment authorized by a guardian or in a situation considered an emergency. Presumably, the U.S. Supreme Court sometime will clarify these discrepancies but has not done so yet. Meanwhile, be *very* cautious (and legal) when insisting that a patient receive ECT or medication against his or her will, even when that patient appears to need it badly. Know your local laws.

Abandonment

Refusing to treat a willing (although possibly difficult) and active patient is to risk the charge of "abandonment." When refusing continued care, always document the reasons (they should be sound, of course), attempt to transfer the patient to another therapist or institution if the patient is willing, make efforts to minimize any risk to the patient (and document), and arrange to care for the patient "in extremis" until the clinical situation has stabilized. Medical cost-containment policies are frequently (typically) not seen as a legitimate reason for terminating care (thus producing a significant and growing problem).

Competency

Psychiatrists are sometimes asked to assess (the court *decides*) whether a patient is mentally competent to perform *specific* functions (e.g., make a will, handle finances, testify in court). Although a judgment for or against competency depends on the context, there are rules for some of these decisions—e.g., to be judged competent to make a will, a person must know (a) that he or she is making a will, (b) the extent and nature of property, and (c) to whom he or she is leaving his or her things. However, to be found incompetent for one task does not necessarily imply incompetence for another (i.e., competency is *task specific*).

CRIMINAL LAW

Competency to Stand Trial

It is held in law that, to receive a fair trial, a person must be able to understand the nature of the charges against him or her, understand the possible penalties, understand legal issues and procedures, and work with his or her attorney and participate rationally in his own defense (*Dusky v United States*). If a person cannot do one or more of these, he or she is "incompetent to stand trial" and usually is transferred to a treatment facility until competency is restored (e.g., medication for a psychosis). Once found competent, the patient is usually returned to court to stand trial. Recently, some states have decided that if a patient's competency cannot be restored in a "reasonable length of time" (e.g., the length of time he or she probably would serve for the crime charged), that patient must continue treatment in a civil facility if committable or be released. Psychiatrists are most commonly the experts asked to help the court decide on competency (the decision is the court's).

Criminal Responsibility

The "not guilty by reason of insanity" plea is much debated by both the legal and psychiatric professions, yet it continues to be used (infrequently) (6). It is *not* widely abused. Part of the general dissatisfaction with this plea centers on whether psychiatrists (or anyone) can retrospectively determine a patient's mental functioning at the time of a crime. Just as an incompetency decision is concerned with the patient's mental state *at the time of the trial*, a responsibility decision involves the mental state *at the time of the crime*. Also in question are the criteria needed to make that judgment. Several different ones are used in different states:

- *The M'Naghten Rule:* Did the person not *know* the nature of his or her act and that it was wrong? This is a common test (one third of states).
- *The Irresistible Impulse Test:* Was a person acting under an "irresistible impulse?" This test is considered unsound alone and is typically combined with other tests.
- *The American Law Institute Test* (ALI Test): Does a person have a mental disease or defect such that he or she "lacks *substantial* capacity either to *appreciate* the criminality of his conduct or to *conform* his conduct to the requirements of the law?" This test adds a "volitional" standard to the "cognitive" standard of the M'Naghten Rule. It is used in approximately one half of the states and in all federal courts.

If one or more of the above conditions are met, the patient may be declared "not guilty by reason of insanity" and be freed of responsibility for his or her crime. If needing treatment at that point, the patient is usually placed in a psychiatric facility until the mental illness remits or until he or she is no longer believed to be a threat to the community because of mental illness.

Many states and the U.S. Congress have considered restrictive modifications (or abolition) of the insanity defense in the wake of the public outcry after John Hinckley's "not guilty" verdict in his shooting of President Reagan. The form the insanity defense ultimately will take is not clear. Leading possibilities appear to be a (a) return to some form of the M'Naghten Rule by eliminating the "volitional" standard and (b) a *guilty but mentally ill* verdict (thus, a person first would be judged and sentenced criminally, then treated in an appropriate setting for mental illness).

PERSONAL ISSUES

Malpractice

The risk that a psychiatrist will be successfully sued for malpractice is low but climbing. Most suits involve use of ECT, improper or inadequately informed use of medication, unusual treatments, sexual involvement with patients, and successful patient suicide (suit brought by relatives). Although it sounds like a platitude, the best defense *is* a strong and respectful therapeutic alliance with the patient. (Yet even that is uncertain protection given a recent successful suit by a father arguing that the therapist had induced false memories of abuse by him in his daughter, the patient.)

Confidentiality

Physicians are ethically obligated to maintain patient confidentiality, except when voluntarily waived by the patient. General knowledge by others of details of a patient's psychiatric treatment or even awareness of psychiatric care can be damaging socially and occupationally to a patient. This requirement for confidentiality continues after the patient's death. Unfortunately, legal protection of the physician for maintaining that confidentiality is far from complete. In some cases, the psychiatrist may be liable if he or she does *not* break privacy; e.g., *Tarasoff v Regents of the University of California* (1976) states that a therapist has a duty to protect a third party threatened harm by the patient (7). This is known as the "*Tarasoff* duty" or "duty to warn." When uncertain, seek consultation from a colleague. Finally, utilization review groups and third-party payers are demanding more privileged information. Become familiar with your own state's laws, because this is legally uncertain ground.

Informed Consent

Informed consent should be sought from all patients for all treatments, but formal (i.e., written) consent should be obtained for physical procedures (e.g., ECT, medication). The patient should be informed about the reasons for the treatment, its nature, the likelihood of success, the dangers and likelihood of side effects, and any alternative treatments.

A major problem arises if the patient is "incapable of being informed" (e.g., due to retardation, OBS, psychosis). A guardian may need to be appointed whose duty would be to make the decision for the patient.

REFERENCES

1. Appelbaum PS, Gutheil TG. *Clinical handbook of psychiatry and the law.* Baltimore: Williams & Wilkins, 1991.
2. Simon RI. *Psychiatry and law for clinicians.* Washington, DC: American Psychiatric Press, 1998.
3. Reid WH, Wise M, Sutton S. The use and reliability of psychiatric diagnosis in forensic settings. *Psychiatr Clin North Am* 1992;15:529–537.
4. McNiel DE, Binder RL. Predictive validity of judgements of dangerousness in emergency civil commitment. *Am J Psychiatry* 1987;144: 197–200.
5. Appelbaum PS. Resurrecting the right to treatment. *Hosp Commun Psychiatry* 1987;38:703–704.
6. Wettstein RM, Mulvey EP, Rogers R. A prospective comparison of four insanity defense standards. *Am J Psychiatry* 1991;148:21–27.
7. Appelbaum PS. Implications of Tarasoff for clinical practice. In: Beck JC, ed. *The potentially violent patient and the Tarasoff decision in psychiatric practice.* Washington, DC: American Psychiatric Press, 1985:10–34.

Subject Index